Amel Ben Hamad
Chiraz Regaieg
Nihed Bouzidi

Maternal-fetal streptococcal B infection

Amel Ben Hamad
Chiraz Regaieg
Nihed Bouzidi

Maternal-fetal streptococcal B infection

Clinical manifestations, treatment and prevention

ScienciaScripts

Imprint

Any brand names and product names mentioned in this book are subject to trademark, brand or patent protection and are trademarks or registered trademarks of their respective holders. The use of brand names, product names, common names, trade names, product descriptions etc. even without a particular marking in this work is in no way to be construed to mean that such names may be regarded as unrestricted in respect of trademark and brand protection legislation and could thus be used by anyone.

Cover image: www.ingimage.com

This book is a translation from the original published under ISBN 978-620-6-72414-8.

Publisher:
Sciencia Scripts
is a trademark of
Dodo Books Indian Ocean Ltd. and OmniScriptum S.R.L publishing group

120 High Road, East Finchley, London, N2 9ED, United Kingdom
Str. Armeneasca 28/1, office 1, Chisinau MD-2012, Republic of Moldova, Europe
Printed at: see last page
ISBN: 978-620-8-16057-9

Table of contents

Introduction

Maternal-fetal infections (MFIs) or early neonatal bacterial infections (EBNIs) are always a concern for all practitioners, due to the severity of certain clinical forms, which can be life-threatening for newborn babies (NNEs), and the difficulties involved in diagnosis. This pathology is widely suspected, but very rarely confirmed (1).

Group B Streptococcus (GBS) or *Streptococcus agalactiae* is a commensal bacterium of the gastrointestinal tract and vagina in women. Vaginal carriage of GBS in women is generally asymptomatic (2). Maternal GBS infection is exceptional (3).

In newborns, Group B Streptococcus is the main etiological agent of early neonatal bacterial infections (4). The main route of transmission is vertical, via the mother's contaminated amniotic and/or vaginal secretions during or just prior to delivery (5). Transmission occurs in 50-75% of cases, and 1-2% of newborns develop a neonatal infection (6).

Today, the worldwide incidence of GBS MFIs has gradually decreased to 0.41 per 1000 live births, thanks to the use of specific preventive measures based on screening for maternal GBS carriage and intrapartum antibiotic prophylaxis (IPP) for colonized women (7,8). However, its incidence remains high in developing countries (9).

Despite therapeutic advances and preventive measures, GBS MFI remains a serious pathology responsible for 150,000 neonatal and infant deaths per year worldwide, with the highest mortality rate in Africa (27%) (7,10); in addition to the risk of neurosensory and cognitive sequelae in GBS meningitis, and even in isolated sepsis (7 to 40%) (11,12).

In Tunisia, GBS screening of pregnant women is not yet routine practice. Few national data are available on GBS MFIs in Tunisia (13,14).

Epidemiology

1 Definitions

Neonatal bacterial infections are divided into neonatal bacterial infections (NBI) or maternal-fetal infections (MFI) or "early onset diseases", and late neonatal infections (LNI) or "late onset diseases".

Precociousness varies from study to study. It occurs between the first 3 and 7 days of life (16,20).

Late neonatal infections occur between 7 and 90 days of age. They are the consequence of postnatal contamination (21).

In our study, only early-onset neonatal infections, occurring within the first 3 days of life, were considered as MFI. We restricted ourselves to the first 72 hours for the following reasons:

-Bacterial infections during this period are exclusively of maternal-fetal origin, with the main germs being GBS and enterobacteria.

-The criteria for initiating ATB treatment are based on maternal and neonatal anamnestic data, as well as clinical and biological data.

-Neonatal infections beyond 72 hours may be due to postnatal contamination.

2 Epidemiology

In industrialized countries, group B streptococci were the main germs responsible for MFIs in full-term babies (22,23).
In a meta-analysis published in 2017, the worldwide incidence of GBS MFI was 0.41 per 1,000 live births (NV): the highest incidence being observed in Africa (between 0.71 and 1.18 per 1,000 NV) and the lowest in Asia (0.32 per 1,000 NV) (9).

In fact, this overall incidence varied from country to country, depending on whether or not certain septicemic infections were taken into account. Definite septicemic infections confirmed by central bacteriological sampling (blood, CSF) were rare, with less than 10% of suspected early infections (9,24,25).

In developing countries, the epidemiology of GBS MFIs remains poorly studied. In several studies, this was explained by the lack of diagnosis of the causes of neonatal morbidity and mortality due to lack of resources (26). In 2015, it was estimated that Africa accounted for 54% of GBS MFI cases worldwide, and 65% of fetal and neonatal deaths (4).

Studies by Scharg (27), Kuhn (28) and Madrid (9) reported an incidence of 0.22 to 0.75 per 1000 NV. In Africa, the incidence of GBS MFI varied between 1.5 and 2 cases per 1000 NV (29).

The study by Stoll et al (23) reported an incidence of 0.4 per 1000 NV of sepsis GBS MFI cases. However, in South Africa, the incidence of septicemic GBS MFI is between 1.5 and 2 cases per 1,000 NV (29).

The following table (Table I) illustrates the differences between countries in the incidence of GBS MFI.

Table I: Incidence of GBS MFIs in the literature

	Authors	*Study period*	*Incidence of septicemic definite MFI (‰ NV)*
In America	*Verani JR (30)*	*2008*	*0.37*
	Nanduri (25)	*2015*	*0.23*
In Europe	*Berardi (Italy) (31)*	*2007*	*0.5*
	Kuhn (France) (28)	*2010*	*0.75*
In Asia	*Madrid (9)*	*2000-2017*	*0.32 (0.22-0.41)*
	Tiskumara (Thailand) (32)	*2009*	*0.14 (0.03-0.4*
In Africa	*Gray et al (33)*	*2007* *2017*	*1.07-2* *0.7*
	Madrid et al (9)	*2000-2017*	*0.71 (0.24-1.18)*
	Sinha et al (34)	*1990-2014*	*1.3 (0.81-1.9)*

MFI: maternal-fetal infection, HC: blood culture, NV: live births

Overall, the incidence of GBS MFIs has fallen considerably over the past fortnight, thanks to widespread screening for genital GBS colonization at the end of pregnancy and per-partum antibiotic prophylaxis for colonized women (30).

In the USA, the incidence of GBS MFIs fell from 1.7 per 1000 births in 1990 to less than 0.35 per 1000 NV in 2008 (30,35). A similar trend was observed in France, where annual incidence fell from 0.69 to 0.23 per 1000 NV between 1997 and 2006 (36).

3-Proportion of MFI with GBS :

GBS remained the most common early invasive pathogen of early neonatal infection, followed by *E coli* (27).

In fact, a prospective study conducted between 2006 and 2009 in America found that GBS remains the most common MFI pathogen, with a prevalence of 43% (23).

Similarly, studies in the Netherlands (21) and Italy (39) also continue to show that GBS is more common *than E coli* in their most recent reporting years (2011 and 2009-2012, respectively).

Pathogenesis

3 Pathogenesis of GBS FMD

Group B Streptococcus or *Streptococcus agalactiae* is a Gram-positive cocci classified by Rebecca Lancefield as group B β-hemolytic streptococci. It is a commensal bacterium of the gastrointestinal tract and vagina in women. In the 1970s, this germ was discovered to be an important pathogen causing invasive bacterial infections in newborn humans during the first week of life. Since then, GBS has been the leading infectious cause of neonatal morbidity and mortality worldwide. Serotypes I, II and especially III are the most common, while IV and V are rarer, and some remain ungroupable (40).

Early neonatal *Streptococcus B* infection begins with asymptomatic colonization of the mother's urogenital tract, followed by transmission of the bacteria to the newborn. Transmission can occur via the blood-borne route, but most often via the ascending route, following contamination of amniotic fluid with ruptured or intact membranes. Inhalation of contaminated maternal vaginal secretions is also possible (21,41). Maternal carriage of GBS and premature rupture of membranes are therefore decisive factors in contamination of the newborn.

Infection is due partly to the bacterium's ability to *adhere to, colonize* and then abnormally *cross the* neonate's epithelial and endothelial barriers, and partly to the immaturity of the immune system, especially in premature infants (42).

The adhesion of *Streptococcus agalactiae* to different cell types is thus a critical step in the tissue invasion required to trigger the infectious process. Bacteria-host cell interactions involve bacterial surface proteins. Some have been identified as ligands for extracellular matrix proteins (fibrinogen or fibronectin), which act as molecular bridges between the bacteria and host cell surface proteins. Other bacterial surface proteins, such as adhesins and pili, promote cell adhesion. Cervical and intestinal epithelial cells can be crossed via cell junctions. The direct cytotoxic action of SGB hemolysin/pigment and the inflammatory reaction also promote the crossing of cell barriers (22). S. agalactiae expresses numerous factors that enable it to counter the host's immune defenses, such as the capsule and C5a peptidase, which interfere with opsonization and modulate the immune and inflammatory response (Figure 20).

Finally, the immaturity of the immune system makes newborns susceptible, particularly in terms of phagocytic functions and the classical and alternative complement pathways (22).

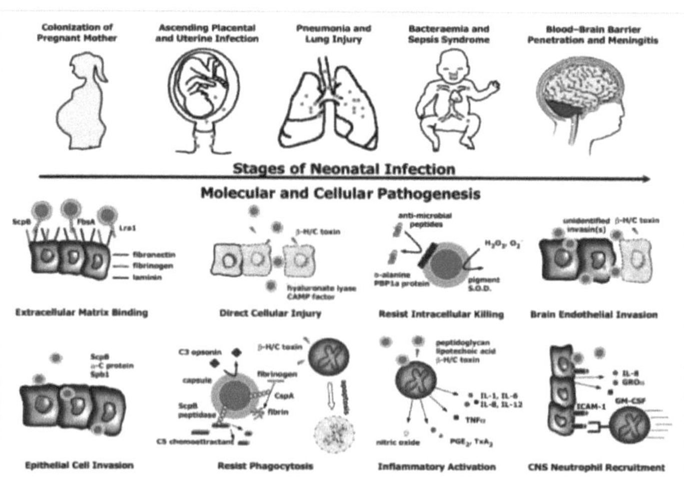

Figure 1: Pathophysiology of early neonatal S. agalactiae infection, after Doran (43)

Maternal characteristics and pregnancy

4 Maternal characteristics

4.1 Maternal age

In the majority of studies, a predominance of young maternal age in GBS MFI has been noted (44-47).

In fact, a retrospective cohort study in the USA, including babies whose mothers had tested negative for GBS, showed that maternal age < 18 years was significantly associated with the risk of GBS MFI ($p<0.001$) (45). This high incidence could be explained by low levels of protective antibodies in the offspring of young mothers, since the latter may be less exposed during their lives to the formation of antibodies specific to the different GBS serotypes (45).

4.2 Parity

According to several authors, primiparity in itself constitutes a risk of GBS MFI (48). This factor could be linked to the young age of the mothers and the often prolonged duration of labor in primiparous women.

4.3 History of GBS infection

A history of neonatal GBS infection was considered a high-risk factor for GBS infection in a subsequent pregnancy. It is this fear of missing out on this infection that has prompted teams to inform and warn the paediatrician and gynaecologist in the event of a history of GBS carriage in a previous pregnancy or a history of a child with a neonatal GBS infection (49) .

4.4 Pregnancy follow-up

Irregular pregnancy follow-up with fewer than 4 perinatal consultations was associated with a high risk of neonatal sepsis (47). In addition, multiple vaginal examinations were associated with a high risk of early neonatal GBS sepsis (50).

4.5 Anamnestic risk factors

The main anamnestic risk factors (RRFs) for GBS MFI found in the literature were known maternal GBS colonization (history of neonatal GBS infection in previous pregnancies, vaginal carriage or GBS bacteriuria in the mother during pregnancy), premature rupture of membranes (RPM $\geq$ 12h), preterm delivery, maternal peripartum fever ($\geq$38°C ; often interpreted as a sign of chorioamniotitis) (51-54). These DRFs were present in 50-75% of GBS MFIs, but their frequency varied from series to series (Table II) (41,55). The infectious history in our study was positive, with one or more of these elements present in 73% of cases.

These risk factors were additive. The presence of more than one factor increased the probability of neonatal infection (52). In fact, Puopolo et al (56) created a score that took into account maternal GBS carriage, intrapartum antibiotic prophylaxis, maternal temperature, gestational age and duration of rupture of membranes to assess the likelihood of GBS MFI in asymptomatic neonates.

Table II: Anamnestic risk factors for GBS FMD in the literature

Author	Cho (57)	Baeringsdottir (41)	Santhanam (50)	Puopolo (56)	Ben Mlik (37)
Year of study	2011 2016	1975-2019	2004-2015	1993 2007	2002 2004
RPM	29%	52%	5.6%	46.4%	59,6%
Maternal carriage of GBS	48.4%	7%	-	35%	-
LA meconial or tinted	9.7%	-	23.8%	-	38,5%
Chorioamniotite	-	9 %	2 %	-	25%
Maternal fever	-	18%	14%	14%	50%
Prematurity	-	25%	14.3%	14%	17,3%

PMR: premature rupture of membranes, AFS: acute fetal distress, AL: amniotic fluid, SGB: Streptococcus B

4.5.1 Maternal colonization with group B Streptococcus

Given the pathogenesis of neonatal GBS infection, vaginal GBS colonization represented a major risk factor for early-onset neonatal GBS disease. For this reason, Disease Control And Prevention Center (CDC) guidelines recommended universal GBS screening of pregnant women at 35 weeks' gestation, with intrapartum antibiotic prophylaxis for carriers (35,58).

Vaginal carriage of GBS in women is generally asymptomatic. According to the literature, the carriage rate varies between 11 and 35% depending on the country, with a worldwide average of 18% (2,4). Maternal GBS infection has been exceptional, with a very low incidence of around 0.38 per 1000 pregnancies (3). Mother-to-child transmission was noted in 40-70% of cases (46,59). In the absence of any intervention, 1-2% of babies born to colonized mothers developed GBS MFIs. This rate varied between 1% and 8% in some early studies (46,59).

In Tunisia, screening for GBS carriage in pregnant women is not yet routine practice. Data on GBS carriage were scarce. A recent study carried out in Tunis between 2014 and 2018 showed a prevalence of GBS vaginal carriage of 12.7% (60). Another cross-sectional study carried out between March and June 2021 in the maternity department of CHU Hédi-Chaker and in private practices in Sfax found a GBS vaginal carriage rate of 27% (54 positive PVs /200 PVs performed) (61).

Nevertheless, vaginal colonization is often transient or intermittent (51), which could confound GBS screening in pregnant women (45), and neonatal GBS disease remains a possibility. This has been reported in several studies (23,62,63). Indeed, sensitivity, specificity, positive predictive value and negative predictive value decreased with increasing delay between the date of PV and the date of delivery (64).

However, a recent prospective study conducted between 2019 and 2020 showed that the risk of GBS MFI in Nborns of GBS-carrying mothers was statistically significant than in those born to GBS-negative women (65).

Maternal GBS bacteriuria ($\geq 10^5$ germs/mL) at any time during pregnancy was a major risk factor for GBS MFI (66). Its prevalence varied according to series from 2 to 7% (30), *which was close to our series (2.2%)*. The risk of developing sepsis in babies born to mothers with a history of urinary tract infection during pregnancy was multiplied by three (47).

4.5.2 Premature rupture of the membranes

Premature rupture of the membranes (PMR) is defined as a spontaneous rupture of the water sac before the onset of labor, and can occur before or at term (59). In 60 to 80% of cases, it occurs beyond 37 weeks' gestation (67). Prolonged opening of the water sac occurs when it lasts $\geq$ 18 hours before birth. However, this threshold varies from author to author (from 24 to 72 hours) (44,59).

It has been well demonstrated in several studies that PMR $\geq$12 hours was associated with a high risk of GBS MFI (50,66,68-70). According to Chan

(59), pregnant women with PMR or prolonged rupture of membranes had a high prevalence of neonatal GBS infection. Puopulo (56) has shown that the risk of MFI increases steadily with the duration of rupture of membranes. It increases by a factor of 2 for a 12-hour rupture and by a factor of 4 for an 18-hour rupture.

4.5.3 Maternal fever and chorioamniotitis

Maternal fever is defined as hyperthermia >38°C. For **chorioamniotitis**, there are several clinical, bacteriological and histological definitions. Avila has shown the uselessness of these different definitions in predicting MFIs, since fever alone should trigger antibiotic therapy in many clinical situations (71).

Puopolo has shown that the risk of early neonatal GBS disease increases as maternal fever rises. This risk was multiplied by 6.5 in the event of intrapartum maternal temperature > 38°C, and by 20 if it exceeded 38.5°C (56,58).

Chorioamniotitis complicated 1 to 3.8% of pregnancies and was associated with increased perinatal morbidity (72,73). It is a major risk factor for early neonatal GBS disease and a cause of antibiotic prophylaxis failure. Its frequency varied (2% to 60%) depending on the series and the definition used (50,57).

Several factors seem to favour the occurrence of chorioamniotitis: RPM > 24 hours, a high number of vaginal touches, prolonged labour of more than 6 hours, maternal colonization with GBS and primiparity (41) .

4.5.4 Prematurity

Prematurity is defined as gestational age < 37 SA (74). MFI is significantly associated with prematurity, and vice versa, prematurity is associated with the risk of MFI (75,76). Immaturity of the immune system and defects in phagocytosis and complement activity explain the increased susceptibility of premature infants to pathogens. In addition, placental transmission of immunoglobulins before 34 days' gestation is not yet optimal, making the potential protection afforded by maternal antibodies to GBS weak (77). Puopolo (56) noted that an increased risk of GBS MFI was associated with both preterm and postterm delivery.

Prematurity in Hoover's series was 28% (78) and Ben Mlik's (37) 23.1%, but in Bahloul's series it was 37.3% (15).

4.5.5 Suspect twin

Twin pregnancy is known to be a predisposing factor for invasive GBS disease (79). The relative risk of infection in the twin of an affected neonate has been calculated to be up to 25-fold. Premature twins are even more susceptible to concomitant infections than their full-term counterparts. The increased susceptibility of twins to GBS infection is probably multifactorial. In early-onset disease, placental invasion by GBS may produce simultaneous perinatal exposures (80). Appearance of amniotic fluid

Meconium amniotic fluid is a historically described risk factor. It has been associated with MFI in some studies (81). However, meconium is no longer included in the criteria for infectious anamnesis in more recent studies.

4.6 Delivery mode

Some authors have reported that Caesarean delivery is significantly associated with GBS MFI, due to the higher rate of Caesarean section in these cases.

In a meta-analysis published in 2017 investigating the risk of early neonatal disease in Nésnés of GBS-colonized pregnant women, scheduled caesarean section before any rupture of membranes was a protective factor against vertical GBS transmission (82). A retrospective cohort study of GBS-negative mothers showed that vaginal delivery was a risk factor for GBS MFI, compared with Caesarean delivery, and the relationship was statistically significant (45). In fact, natural childbirth may favor the passage of GBS into the maternal genital tract. However, Caesarean section does not prevent maternal-fetal transmission of GBS, as it can occur through intact amniotic membranes (46).

Boyer et al (70) showed that there was no significant difference between vaginal and caesarean deliveries, although there was a higher rate of GBS IMF in caesarean births. This could be explained by the fact that Caesarean sections were indicated for complications of labour, most often due to infectious causes.

Neonatal characteristics

5 Characteristics of newborns at birth
5.1 Term

Premature newborns are more susceptible to bacterial infections, given the immaturity of the immune system (83). Indeed, prematurity was considered not only a risk factor for MFI, but also a sign of fetal infection, because fetal infection is a cause of prematurity, particularly for terms less than 34 SA (84). However, infection of the premature baby does not differ fundamentally from that of the term baby, but rather in frequency and severity. Infection of premature babies has been found in several series at high rates. Fluegge et al (85) reported that prematurity was present in 22.4% of GBS MFI cases, which was close to our results (22.6% of cases).

In 2011, Weston (84) noted that prematurity was more likely to be associated with Escherichia coli MFIs (39%), and that GBS accounted for only 26.4% of germs versus 45.4% in the term-born.

GBS remains the predominant germ of MFI in term newborns (27).

5.2 Gender

A clear male predominance has been reported in various series in the literature (68,87,88), with male frequency ranging from 66.6% to 55.9%.

5.3 Birth weight

Low birth weight is a classic factor in GBS MFI (23,44,55). In a systemic review published in 2014, the authors showed that very low-birth-weight Nés had a higher risk of GBS MFI (up to 3%) and mortality of up to 30%, even with immediate antibiotic therapy (89).

In the Tunisian series, this population represented between 21 and 33% of GBS FMIs (37,86). In other series, the rate of low-birth-weight babies was much higher, ranging from 40 to 68% (23,47,75,90). This could be explained by the high percentage of premature babies.

5.4 Apgar score

Jackson (91) has suggested that poor adaptation to life outside the womb, with recourse to heavy resuscitation in the delivery room, apart from obstetric causes, should be considered a sign of early neonatal infection. Other studies have noted that a low Apgar score is associated with a higher risk of neonatal sepsis (92)....

Clinical picture

6 Clinical study
6.1 Age of onset of clinical signs

Clinical signs of GBS-MFI often begin within the first 24 hours of life (9,44,55,58,70,93). Zaleznik DF (94) showed that GBS MFI presented in 60-70% of cases before H24 of life, 32% between H24 and 48 of life and 8% of cases after 48 hours of life.

Bromberger added that intrapartum antibiotic prophylaxis did not delay the onset of clinical signs (95). Indeed, all term babies exposed to IPA developed symptoms in 95% of cases before 24 hours of life in cases of GBS MFI (9,55).

6.2 Clinical signs

Clinical diagnosis is difficult, as symptoms are polymorphic and not specific to GBS (96,97). The early onset of symptoms at birth or in the first few hours of life, in the form of respiratory disorders with or without radiological pneumopathy, hemodynamic disorders and rarely pulmonary arterial hypertension (PAH), characterizes GBS IMF (98).

In the literature, the majority of GBS MFI cases are symptomatic. The main symptoms are respiratory distress, refusal to suckle, early jaundice and fever (99,100).

Neonatal respiratory distress (NRD) is the typical presentation of GBS MFI (41,87). Andersen and Baeringsdottir (41,101) found respiratory distress in 72% and 80% of GBS MFIs respectively. Polypnoea may be the sole manifestation of sepsis with or without pneumonia (96). In premature infants, MFI may manifest as apnea (41). Infection may also simulate or be associated with hyaline membrane disease (41).

DRNN may be complicated by **refractory hypoxemia** resulting from PAH.

It may or may not be associated with radiographic lung parenchymal abnormalities. Pathogenically, the release of endothelins and cytokines by GBS causes pulmonary hypertension in newborns. In addition, phosphatidylglycerol and cardiolipin, the membrane phospholipids of GBS, are most associated with PAH (43). Diagnosis is based on cardiac ultrasound, which confirms the high level of pulmonary resistance. In the absence of specific treatment (nitric oxide, hyperventilation, antibiotic therapy), the course is critical.

Full-term babies are more susceptible to **fever** in cases of severe sepsis, pneumonia and meningitis, while premature babies are more susceptible to **hypothermia**, particularly during the first 48 h of life (96).

Neurological signs included impaired reactivity, convulsions, tonus abnormalities, poor contact and dissociated archaic reflexes. These signs, in a clinico-biological context of sepsis, were suggestive of meningitis.

6.3 Clinical forms

In 2019, De Gier et al (102) showed the predominance of sepsis and pneumonia in early neonatal GBS disease and the relative rarity of meningitis (Table III).

Author (Reference)	Carlough (103)	Heath (44)	Baeringsdottir (41)	Ji (104)	Madrid (9)	Joubrel (55)
Sepsis	69%	69%	100%	83.6%	78%	61%
Pneumonia	26%	26%	27%	52.1%	-	6%
Meningitis	11%	11%	11%	12.3%	16%	27%

6.3.1 Sepsis

Sepsis is the main clinical form of GBS MFI. It is defined as an invasive bacterial infection of the blood, which may have other secondary localizations, notably meningeal and pulmonary (84). Failure to isolate GBS in a central bacteriological specimen does not rule out sepsis (105). For this reason, there was no uniform, consensual definition of neonatal sepsis (105,106). In 2012, the National Institute for Health and Care Excellence (NICE) recommended the diagnosis of "culture-negative sepsis" in the face of symptomatic infection with no identified bacterial cause (107). The latter suggested the presence of revealing symptoms and/or a CRP ≥ 25 mg/L and the presence of GBS in the mother's vaginal/rectal swab or in peripheral swabs in the neonate. The initiation of antibiotic therapy in the newborn could be an additional criterion(108).

Joubrel (55) showed that early neonatal GBS infection was associated with sepsis (61%), while late neonatal GBS infection was associated with meningitis *(55%)*.

Symptoms of neonatal sepsis can range from non-specific signs to full-blown hemodynamic collapse(93). Initial symptoms may include irritability, lethargy or refusal to suckle. Some patients rapidly develop respiratory distress, fever, hypothermia or even shock (30,44).

Infected newborns are sometimes initially asymptomatic, a situation that should not delay antibiotic therapy if the history is suggestive. In fact, symptoms may be absent or discreet, especially in the case of maternal antibiotic therapy (13). These discrete signs have been represented by recently added markers: an abnormal heart rate profile with loss of variability, transient decelerations (109) and oxygen saturation < 95% before 12 h of life and without improvement 2 h later (110,111). These discrete signs of MFI may be intricate and difficult to differentiate from physiological phenomena induced by cardiorespiratory adaptation to extrauterine life. This underlines the importance of proper interpretation of any clinical sign of secondary onset in neonates.

This could be explained by difficulties or limitations in the punctual assessment of probable discrete clinical signs. The hypothesis that the use of AIP could mask sepsis, due to the prenatal transfer of antibiotics rendering the blood cultures of the neonates negative, was quickly eliminated. In fact, the mothers of these patients had not received AIP. Moreover, these babies could be treated in time before the onset of clinical signs.

6.3.2 Pneumonia

Respiratory distress of infectious origin reflects lung parenchymal damage. It is secondary to lung cell damage, due in part to the cytotoxic properties of GBS hemolysin and the influx of neutrophils (112). Inhalation of amniotic fluid leads to colonization of the respiratory mucosa, rapidly followed by the development of pneumonia. Clinical expression includes polypnoea, signs of struggle +/- hypoxemia. Diagnosis also requires a chest X-ray compatible with the appearance of infectious alveolitis.

6.3.3 Meningitis

GBS is the dominant cause of neonatal meningitis, accounting for 77% of MFI cases with meningeal localization (113). According to Lin (114), serotype III was responsible for more than half of all GBS meningitis cases.

The lack of specificity of clinical signs in newborns makes diagnosis difficult(115). Meningeal involvement is often revealed by fever and/or neurological signs (reactivity disorders, convulsions, tonus abnormalities, bulging fontanelle), which require lumbar puncture (34).

In Bahloul's (15) study of GBS MFI, which included 75 cases, 5 cases of neonatal meningitis were diagnosed. Thus, the rate of meningitis in neonates with GBS MFI was 6.6%. This could be explained by an underestimation of the incidence of early GBS meningitis due to delayed lumbar punctures in view of the clinical instability of the neonates.

In the literature, the incidence of early GBS meningitis fell significantly with the use of AIP, while the incidence of late meningitis remained stable (116,117). In France, the incidence of early GBS meningitis decreased significantly from 0.06 (95% CI, 0.04 to 0.08) to 0.02 (95% CI, 0.01 to 0.04) from 2001 to 2014 (117).

In total, clinical forms of GBS MFI can be classified as isolated sepsis, sepsis with meningitis, sepsis with pneumonia or sepsis with meningitis and pneumonia (41).

Further tests

7 Further tests

7.1 Biological tests

Newborns with GBS MFI may initially be asymptomatic. For this reason, biological tests are essential in the presence of any suspected GBS infection (118).

7.1.1 Complete blood count (CBC)

The interpretation of CBC in neonates is complex. It must take account of physiological variations according to gestational age, mode of delivery and sampling site (118).

In neonatal infection, all three lineages can be affected. The most specific hematological signs during neonatal infection were, in chronological order, leukopenia, neutropenia, myelemia and hyperleukocytosis (119).

Leukopenia is an important sign of GBS MFI (120). It was more associated with infection than **hyperleukocytosis** (121). Hornik et al showed that neutropenia was a better marker of sepsis and was often correlated with vital prognosis (119). However, early leukopenia occurring at the very first clinical signs was often overlooked if samples were not systematically repeated (122).

Thrombocytopenia is a late and unspecific sign of infection. It was most frequently observed in severe forms (99,123).

Anemia is frequently seen in infected newborns. Its rapid onset, often associated with jaundice, suggests a hemolytic mechanism. However, it is an unspecific sign of infection. A few studies have noted that anemia is a risk factor for early neonatal sepsis (124).

7.1.2 C-reactive protein (CRP)

In the presence of infection, macrophage release of pro-inflammatory cytokines induces hepatic synthesis of pro-inflammatory proteins, including C-reactive protein (CRP). A globulin synthesized by the liver, CRP does not cross the placental barrier. Virtually undetectable at birth (~ 0.1 mg/L), its physiological concentration rises to reach a maximum between H24 and H36. The upper normal limit is very close to 10 mg/L (125). In the case of infection, a delay of 6 to 12 hours was observed between the start of the infectious process and the increase in CRP, which could explain the possibility of false negatives in the case of sampling at birth (96,126,127). CRP is the most widely used parameter for the diagnosis of MFI. It is widely available and its determination is simple, rapid and economical (125,128).

Its sensitivity and specificity in cases of MFI were of the order of 65.6% and 83% respectively on the first two determinations (129,130). Andersen (101) found that CRP increased after more than 12 hours of symptoms in 82% of GBS MFI cases.

In addition, several studies (129,131) have shown that the negative predictive value (NPV) of two successive determinations is greater than 90%, enabling antibiotic therapy to be neither started nor stopped. Sequential CRP determination between 24 and 48 hours after the onset of clinical signs increases its sensitivity for the diagnosis of neonatal sepsis (128). In addition, serial CRP is used to monitor response to treatment in infected neonates (132).

In cases of early GBS meningitis, CRP may be a good indicator. It was consistently positive in the Philips series (133).

However, several factors can increase CRP levels, such as inhalation of meconium fluid, traumatic or ischemic tissue damage, chorioamniotitis and hemolysis (134).

Several studies have shown that CRP is a good prognostic indicator of neonatal sepsis (99,135). Li et al have shown that elevated CRP is a predictor of the severity of neonatal sepsis (135).

7.1.3 Procalcitonin (PCT)

Procalcitonin is an important biomarker of early neonatal sepsis. It is increasingly used in neonates (136). PCT, like CRP, does not cross the placenta, and is therefore unaffected by maternal fever during labor (137). It is synthesized by monocytes and hepatocytes. PCT elevation begins 4 to 6 hours after exposure to the bacterial germ (126). This more rapid response than CRP makes PCT an attractive alternative to CRP for the detection of MFI (96,138,139).

The sensitivity and specificity of PCT appear to be better than those of CRP in definite MFI: sensitivity 82% versus 73% and specificity 95% versus 83% (129,140,141). Its negative predictive value was estimated at 93%, enabling bacterial infection to be ruled out in neonates (142).

However, PCT exhibits a number of physiological variations, with a marked physiological rise and fall during the first 72 hours of life, making interpretation of these values difficult. For this reason, the majority of international recommendations retain the PCT assay primarily for the early diagnosis of late neonatal infections, in order to distinguish bacterial from viral infections (143).

In addition, other perinatal factors, such as chorioamniotitis, prolonged PMR, perinatal asphyxia and maternal preeclampsia, may increase CRP and PCT values (138,140).

All in all, CRP, combined with a blood count, is the most widely used combination. PCT has an interesting role to play in the early diagnosis of

MFIs, particularly at the cord, but also in the diagnosis of nosocomial infections (142).

However, biological abnormalities are not specific to the causative agent.

7.2 Bacteriological tests

In the absence of valid clinical criteria and biomarkers, a positive microbial culture from a normally sterile site (blood, cerebrospinal fluid) is the "gold standard" for defining neonatal sepsis (142).

7.2.1 Blood culture

Blood culture is the reference test for the definitive diagnosis of MFI. Blood cultures are not routinely taken in all neonates suspected of having MFI. It is indicated prior to the initiation of any empirical antibiotic therapy in newborns (142,144).

Guerti et al (145) have shown that the time to positivity of neonatal blood cultures differs significantly according to germ type. Moreover, these authors noted that sensitivities for Gram-positive bacteremia after an incubation time of 24, 48 and 72 hours were 51, 87 and 96% respectively. This finding was similar to that of Kumar et al (146): they noted that a 48-hour period was sufficient to exclude sepsis in asymptomatic neonates, and a 72-hour incubation period was sufficient to detect all clinically important infections using bacterial culture.

For GBS, the time to positivity of a blood culture was 36 hours in 96 to 100% of cases. (147-149).

However, microbial cultures suffer from low sensitivity.

This low sensitivity of blood cultures could be explained by :

- Too small a volume of blood sampled, less than 1 mL. Indeed, Connell noted that blood cultures with adequate volume were twice as likely to give a positive result (150).

Therefore, a minimum volume of at least 1% of blood mass (=0.8 mL/kg) is recommended, which is not always possible (63) ;

- The intermittent nature of bacteremia means that blood cultures must be repeated (151) ;
- AIP: According to Dagnew AF (152), the use of antibiotic prophylaxis in pregnant women colonized with GBS, particularly when incomplete, may not be sufficient to prevent clinical neonatal infection, but may inhibit GBS growth in blood and CSF cultures. Other studies had shown that AIP did not appear to delay the time to blood culture positivity (153).

7.2.2 Lumbar puncture

Bacteriological examination of cerebrospinal fluid (CSF) confirms the diagnosis of GBS meningitis, the most dreaded complication of neonatal infection.

The value of systematic lumbar puncture (LP) in the initial assessment of suspected MFI in neonates remains controversial (154). Lumbar puncture is essential immediately in the event of deterioration in general condition (severe sepsis or severe respiratory disorders) or neurological signs, and after stabilization of clinical condition in order to tolerate the procedure (46,155,156). In addition, it is recommended to perform the procedure secondarily if the blood culture is positive, "the main risk factor for meningitis" (126). However, a negative blood culture does not rule out the diagnosis of meningitis, as blood cultures can be negative in up to 38% of newborns with meningitis (154,158).

Some authors have indicated LP in cases of significant inflammatory syndrome (151). However, no CRP threshold has been defined, but its elevation is proportional to the duration of the infectious syndrome. An elevated CRP of over 60-80 mg/L indicates a long delay between the onset of the infectious process and the first sample, and theoretically increases the risk of meningeal localization (151). Furthermore, CRP elevation above a certain threshold is no longer an indication for LP (63,159).

Interpretation of LP results is sometimes difficult, as diagnosis relies on the results of CSF culture, which is associated with high false-negative rates (115,160). This may be explained by the fact that group B streptococci have been shown to disappear from the CSF after eight hours of appropriate antibiotics (161).

In these situations, it is important to interpret the cytological and biochemical parameters of the CSF (cell count, glycorrhachia and proteinorrhachia) in order to make a presumptive diagnosis of meningitis (162). Indeed, the diagnosis of neonatal meningitis can be made on the basis of an initial positive blood culture and if the CSF cytobiochemical study is abnormal after 24 to 36 h of prior antibiotic therapy (156). However, it has been shown in several studies that many factors alter the standards of interpretation of CSF parameters, including gestational age, postnatal age and traumatic LP (154,155,163).

Low glucose and high protein concentrations in CSF are markers with high specificity for the diagnosis of meningitis (63).

Bonadio et al (164) noted that in infected term newborns, a WBC count > 20 - 30 cells/mm^3 corresponded to meningeal inflammation, making the diagnosis of bacterial meningitis probable. For Garges (154), a leukocyte count of more than 20 - 25 cells/mm^3 in the CSF of term newborns was considered abnormal. The sensitivity of this value was 79% and its specificity 81% for diagnosing bacterial neonatal meningitis.

On the other hand, a positive culture may be observed in bacterial meningitis despite a normal CSF leukocyte count (154,165). Recently, Zurina et al (115) showed that 13% of confirmed cases of meningitis had a normal CSF WBC count.

In recent years, it has been demonstrated that **polymerase chain reaction (PCR)** analysis of CSF can be useful in confirming the diagnosis of bacterial meningitis (162) . PCR is a rapid and accurate method for diagnosing meningitis in neonates. It has high sensitivity and specificity, even in neonates who have received antibiotic therapy (115,162).

7.2.3 Peripheral sampling

Peripheral swabs (PS) are bacteriological samples taken from various peripheral sites. The most commonly used are gastric, auricular, rectal, oropharyngeal, mucocutaneous, umbilical and sometimes placental swabs.

Easy to perform, the interpretation of PP is often tricky due to the frequency of GBS colonization (142).

Gastric fluid culture can only be interpreted in the first 4 to 6 hours of life. Gram staining of gastric fluid is positive only when the bacterial concentration is $\geq 10^5$ colonies/ml; its negativity therefore does not prejudge the result of the culture; despite this, its NPV is excellent. If positive, it only reflects antenatal colonization of the amniotic fluid and does not prejudge infection (151). Gastric aspiration was considered one of the most widely used PP for the diagnosis of MFI. For Aujard Y (151), the low sensitivity of blood cultures and the worrying trend in bacterial resistance, particularly to enterobacteria, justify maintaining gastric sampling in cases of suspected MFI, particularly in premature infants. Gastric sampling is the only way of keeping a bacterial epidemiological watch, and knowledge of this is the basis for the choice of first-line, probabilistic antibiotic therapy. It also enables treatment to be adapted in the event of a resistant strain (151). However, gastric sampling is no longer recommended (121,137,166,167).

Wang (136) tested oropharyngeal secretions from premature infants, tracheal secretions and gastric swabs for GBS and showed that PP may well reflect the state of GBS colonization. However, Gerdes (168) and Jost C (142) have demonstrated their limited value for the diagnosis of MFI. Skin sampling is only indicated in the event of a visible lesion.

Placental smears are useful in cases of macroscopic placental lesions.

Bacteriological examination of tracheal aspirates can be useful if obtained immediately and sterilely after placement of the intratracheal tube. For a neonate intubated for several days, tracheal aspirates are of no value in the diagnosis of MFI (63).

Thus, publications by the CDC in 2010, the **American Academy of Pediatrics (AAP)** in 2011 and the Swiss Society of Neonatology in 2013 no longer recommend peripheral sampling (121,169).

7.2.4 Antibiotic sensitivity

In the literature, all isolates tested were sensitive to penicillin, ampicillin and vancomycin (170,171).

Indeed, Dahesh S et al (170) reported that despite the increasing use of antibiotics, group B streptococci remained susceptible to penicillin as well as to most B-Lactams, and penicillin remained the first-line antibiotic for preventing and treating early GBS MFI.

However, since 2008, strains of GBS with reduced susceptibility to penicillin have been reported(171,172). Indeed, very rare isolates recently identified with reduced susceptibility to penicillin have been reported in Japan and the USA(^). A point mutation in the GBS *pbp* 2x gene has been identified as a possible explanation for this reduced sensitivity(170,173).

Recent studies have also reported an increase in the prevalence of resistance to other antibiotics among GBS isolates, particularly macrolides(174). These findings were comparable to the Phares series (20), which showed that 32% of isolates were resistant to erythromycin, clindamycin or both.

Similarly, in the Back EE series (174), resistance rates to both erythromycin and clindamycin were 50.7% and 38.4%, respectively. A study carried out in the USA between 1999 and 2005 (20) concluded that virtually all isolates (99%) that were resistant to clindamycin were also resistant to erythromycin, and that erythromycin resistance was highest among serotype V isolates compared with other serotypes. In the series by Kharrat (61), which studied the serotypes of neonatal GBS infections, macrolide resistance was greater for serotype V strains (P=0.024).

Recent epidemiological data from Canada, China and Portugal have reported the emergence of a multidrug-resistant sublineage of CC17 GBS with acquired resistance to 4 classes of antimicrobials: tetracyclines, aminoglycosides, macrolides and lincosamides (lincomycins, clindamycins) (173,175).

According to Hayes K (173), several countries have noted increased resistance rates in recent years. In addition, resistance to other classes of antibiotics, such as the Fluoroquinolones, also continued to rise.

7.2.5 Other bacteriological samples

Urine cytobacteriological examination (UCE) is not indicated for early sepsis less than 72 hours old (137).

The diagnosis of neonatal infections is likely to benefit from new molecular methods, in particular universal **polymerase chain reaction (PCR)** or multiplex PCR. This new technique is currently considered a better tool for identifying sepsis and the causative germ more rapidly than blood culture (176) .

A Cochrane review published in 2017 (177) and a study carried out in

London published in 2020 (127) showed that PCR, a highly valuable technique, is a possible means of diagnosing neonatal infection, essentially in Nborns where cultures were negative. PCR tests had a sensitivity of over 90% with a specificity of 99%, which was around 13% higher than blood cultures (93).

7.2.6 Bacteriological features of GBS

Streptococcus B is a capsulated bacterium that appears as a Gram-positive cocci, diplococcus or short chain.

There are currently ten serotypes: Ia, Ib, II, III, IV, V, VI, VII, VIII, IX. The most common serotypes in MFI are III (60.6%) and Ia (17.3%) (40).

This classification into serotypes can be refined by searching for c, R and X wall proteins. Thanks to more advanced molecular methods such as multilocus sequence typing (MLST), GBS has been classified into several sequence types (ST) and clonal complexes (CC) according to their genetic relatedness (41).

The capsule is a major virulence factor and an important target for vaccine formulations currently under development. The distribution of GBS serotypes varies with population and geographic location (144). For Edmond et al (178), serotype III (48.9%) was the most frequently identified serotype in GBS MFI, followed by serotypes Ia (22.9%), Ib (7%), II (6.2%) and V (9.1%). In the USA, the most frequent serotypes were Ia (30%), III (28%), V (18%) and II (13%) (20).

In a study conducted at CHU Hedi Chaker between 2012 and 2020, involving 45 strains isolated from early neonatal Streptococcus B infection, serotype V was dominant (31.1%) followed by serotype III in 28.9%, serotype II in 17.8% and serotype IV in 6.7% (61).

Several studies (179,180) have shown that type III is associated with the majority of complicated neonatal infections, especially meningitis.

Furthermore, it has been shown that the ST-17 sequence type is strongly associated with neonatal meningitis, hence the term "hypervirulent" strain (21,181).

7.3 Other paraclinical examinations :

❖ **Chest X-ray**

The various radiological aspects of GBS MFI have been well studied in the literature (182,183). Chest radiography is suggestive of infection in the presence of micro-macro nodular opacities or a systematized focus. However, pulmonary infection or the pulmonary localization of GBS MFI can take on all the radiological aspects of other etiologies of respiratory distress (182,184).

A normal chest X-ray in the presence of respiratory distress does not rule out pulmonary infection.

❖ **Lung ultrasound**

Lung ultrasound is becoming an increasingly common examination in neonatology (185). It is a non-irradiating, high-performance and easily accessible diagnostic tool. In neonates, specific ultrasound findings have been described for the diagnosis of pleurisy, pneumothorax, hyaline membrane disease, meconium inhalation and infectious alveolitis. Today, lung ultrasound is an interesting tool to help clinicians make therapeutic decisions at birth (185).

Therapeutic management

8 Therapeutic management

Apart from symptomatic treatment of respiratory and/or hemodynamic distress, treatment of MFIs is essentially based on appropriate antibiotic therapy. Antibiotic therapy in the neonatal period is a special case, due to the non-specificity of bacterial infection criteria, variable epidemiological data, age-specific pharmacokinetic parameters and the sometimes rapidly evolving nature of certain severe infections (186).

8.1 Antibiotic therapy

Bearing in mind, on the one hand, the fear of failing to treat early neonatal infection in time and, on the other, the adverse effects of antibiotics in a large number of babies with suspected infection, we feel it necessary to carefully study the indications for antibiotic therapy in cases of suspected GBS IMF.

8.1.1 Indications for antibiotic therapy

The therapeutic strategy for the management of MFI varies from one country to another, and even from one team to another in the same country.

Authors from all over the world (64,109,140) recommend that all symptomatic neonates should be treated with intravenous probabilistic TBA as a matter of urgency, after a biological and bacteriological work-up, as they are "until proven otherwise" suspected of early neonatal infection (188-190). The problem lay with asymptomatic newborns. Indications for antibiotic therapy remain controversial (18).

In the meantime, the AAP, the CDC and the Société Française de Néonatologie (SFN) have recommended immediate treatment of asymptomatic ("well-appearing") full-term or premature babies born at high risk of infection (in the context of chorioamniotitis or maternal fever) (137,191,192).

In 2017, the Société Française de Néonatologie (SFN) updated these recommendations. It advocated limiting further investigations and reducing the use of broad-spectrum probabilistic antibiotic therapy in low-risk MFI situations in favor of close monitoring (72). **In 2018,** the first MFI management protocol was developed in Tunisia. This protocol was the subject of a multicenter study. It was used in the 4 level III maternity centers: CHU Hedi Chaker Sfax, CHU Farhat Hached Sousse, Tunis Military Hospital and Monastir Maternity and Neonatology Center. It was subsequently validated by the 4 neonatology teams who participated in this study (Appendix 3) (19). The authors opted not to treat asymptomatic neonates with term > 34SA whose mothers had received adequate antibiotic prophylaxis, irrespective of their infectious history (group A). In the case of inadequate antibiotic prophylaxis, antibiotic therapy is indicated as soon as a positive CRP > 10mg/L is detected in high-risk newborns (group B). All newborns who become symptomatic (group C) should receive antibiotic therapy after HC. This protocol is similar to others currently used in the literature (109,125,140).

At the end of our study, we should be vigilant in the event of chorioamniotitis or RPM >12 hours, even if the neonate is asymptomatic, bearing in mind that in our local conditions systematic screening for GBS and maternal antibiotic prophylaxis are not yet routine practice. This is to avoid missing out on a definite GBS FMD.

However, systematic antibiotic therapy is no longer indicated for asymptomatic newborns. Antibiotic use has undesirable effects: it disturbs the normal digestive flora, leading to the emergence of multi-resistant germs, especially in premature babies. These germs can be a source of hospital infection, necrotizing enterocolitis and death. Similarly, prolonged use of $3^{\text{ème}}$ generation cephalosporins (Cefotaxime) is a risk factor for invasive candidiasis. In addition, it disrupts the bacterial ecosystem in neonatal care units, with low-noise progression of bacterial resistance(63).

8.1.2 Choice of antibiotic therapy

Although the bacterial epidemiology of MFIs has changed since the era of antibiotic prophylaxis, GBS remains the most common germ in term and near-term neonates (40-45% of cases), followed by TEscherichia coli (10-15% of cases) (23,27,84).

Antibiotic susceptibility studies point us in the direction of first-line antibiotic therapy. Ampicillin combined with an aminoglycoside covers the main pathogens associated with early neonatal sepsis. This combination is effective against *Streptococcus Agalatiae,* most *other Streptococcus species, Enterococci* and *Lesteria monocytogenes*, although listeria infection is rare in pregnancy (121). Although two-thirds of E. coli strains and most other gram-negative bacilli (GNB) are resistant to ampicillin, the majority remain sensitive to gentamicin in 96% of cases(23). However, aminoglycosides alone are inactive against GBS. This is low-level natural resistance.

The SFN recommends the combination of Ampicillin + Gentamycin in cases of *Streptococcus agalactiae-positive* blood cultures (189,194). Similarly, the AAP, CDC and ANAES recommend the combination of Ampicillin + Gentamicin in cases of suspected MFI, pending culture results and antibiotic susceptibility testing (137,156,189). Combination with an aminoglycoside is necessary for a synergistic bactericidal effect. The results of our study support these recommendations, since all GBS isolates tested were sensitive to Ampicillin.

The combination of a $3^{\text{ème}}$ generation cephalosporin (C3G) is justified in cases of severe disease (121) and meningeal localization. Cefotaxime in sufficient doses is the recommended C3G, given its efficacy against GBS, absence of resistance and good diffusion in the CSF (63). The use of ceftriaxone in neonates as part of the management of GBS MFI is contraindicated (194).

In cases of neonatal meningitis, some teams recommend "preventive" treatment of intracerebral complications with Ciprofloxacin. In cases of GBS, Rifampicin, whose intrinsic anti-inflammatory and pharmacodynamic properties are equivalent to those of ciprofloxacin, has been proposed for its better antibiotic activity against Gram-positive cocci, including GBS, but has never been evaluated (195).

When GBS is isolated by blood culture, lumbar puncture should be performed if not previously done, and antibiotic therapy adjusted according to the results of CSF and HC analysis, using the narrowest spectrum of appropriate antibiotics (107,121,137,169).

8.1.3 Duration and dosage of antibiotic therapy

The duration of treatment depends on the location of the GBS infection. It varies from author to author.

The Société Française de néonatologie recommends Ampicillin 100 mg/kg/d in 2 injections **for 7 days**, combined with Gentamicin for **2 days,** in the case of GBS bacteremia and in the absence of meningeal localization**.** In cases of GBS meningitis, Gentamicin is given for **2 to 5 days**, followed by Ampicillin 200 mg/kg/d in 2 injections up to 7 days of age, then Ampicillin 200 mg/kg/d in 3 injections for a total treatment period of **14 days** in cases with an immediately favorable outcome (194**).**

For the AAP and CDC, GBS sepsis without meningeal involvement is treated for 10 days, and GBS meningitis is treated for at least 14 days (63). NICE (107) indicates that the duration of TBA in the case of MFI with positive blood cultures, or in the case of strong suspicion of sepsis but negative blood cultures, should be 7 days.

In observational studies, neonates with culture-negative sepsis were generally treated for 5 to 7 days, and mortality was very low (196).

Fjalstad (197) found a median treatment time of 8 days for confirmed MFIs and 5 to 7 days for HC-negative MFIs.

Labenne et al. (196), or excessive treatment duration was observed in only 28% of cases.

Due to ototoxicity and nephrotoxicity, Aminoside is generally discontinued after 2 to 3 days of treatment, and in cases of meningitis, it is continued for up to 5ème days (107).

Antibiotic dosages should be adjusted according to gestational age, post-natal age and weight.

The intravenous (IV) route is the only one recommended. It must be performed rigorously (18,186). The intramuscular (IM) route is strongly discouraged because of its toxic local effects and pain. It is acceptable only in exceptional cases, such as when the IV route is temporarily unavailable (18). Oral relays are not recommended for infections confirmed by blood culture or CSF (194).

8.2 Symptomatic treatment

Symptomatic treatment should be started at the same time as antibiotic therapy. Its aim is to maintain homeostasis of the internal environment and correct metabolic disorders. The main symptomatic measures include maintaining core temperature by placing the neonate in an incubator, correcting metabolic disorders such as acidosis and hypoglycemia, which are frequent in neonatal infections, and monitoring respiratory and neurological hemodynamics. Thus, in the event of septic shock, treatment calls first for vascular filling to restore effective blood volume, followed by inotropes if necessary. Noradrenaline is particularly indicated in septic shock. Hydrocortisone may be combined with the above measures, particularly in cases of refractory shock and/or suspected adrenal insufficiency (198).

Respiratory function control: respiratory distress is frequent and severe in GBS MFIs (41). Treatment can range from simple oxygen therapy to assisted ventilation.

Evolution

9 Evolution

9.1 Neonatal mortality

Despite advances in neonatal resuscitation, early antibiotic therapy and improved prophylactic measures, the prognosis for GBS MFI remains poor. Mortality due to this neonatal pathology remains a global public health problem (4).

The rate of neonatal mortality due to GBS MFIs has fallen sharply over the years. Currently, GBS-MFI mortality ranges from 4 to 7% in developed countries, and from 17 to 37% in Africa (9).

The global rate advanced in 2017 is (8.4%) so it was lower than that reported in the African series (Table IV).

Table IV: Mortality rates in GBS septicemic IMF

Authors	*Stoll (23)*	*Vergadi (199)*	*Joubrel (55)*	*Bahloul (15)*
Study period	*2006-2009*	*1995-2016*	*2015*	*2008-2010*
Country	*America*	*America*	*France*	*Tunisia*
Mortality rate	*16%*	*6.2%*	*10%*	*10%*

Death rates varied according to the samples studied (term, year of study, etc.). As indicated in recent studies, several factors could explain the reduction in mortality rates, including antibiotic prophylaxis for mothers and antibiotic therapy for at-risk newborns, and improved management of critically ill newborns (114).

9.2 Risk factors associated with mortality

In the literature, the main factors associated with mortality were

prematurity, low birth weight, severe respiratory distress and meningitis

(55,200).

9.2.1 Prematurity:

The lower the gestational age, the higher the neonatal mortality. Its prevalence was 10 to 15 times higher in premature than in term babies (103).

In a study carried out between 1999 and 2005 in the United States, Phares et al (20) found a case-fatality rate of 20 to 30% in infants under 33 weeks' gestation, versus 2 to 3% in full-term infants. Similarly, Weston et al (84) found that the GBS-MFI mortality rate was lower in the term newborn (0-2%) than in premature newborns (22-30%).

More recent studies have shown similar results. Hoover et al (78) reported in a study published in 2020 that preterm newborns (<37SA) with GBS MFI had a mortality rate of 19%, compared with 2% in full-term newborns. However, it has been estimated that the mortality rate among very premature infants with a gestational age < 33 weeks may be as high as 30% (201). .

9.2.2 Low birth weight

Mortality due to FMF varies significantly according to term and therefore birth weight. It was higher in low-birth-weight infants (27,55).

Joubrel (55) showed that low birth weight was the most important mortality factor. Low-birth-weight infants (<2500g) hospitalized for GBS MFI had a higher mortality rate than those with a birth weight above 2500g (OR=3.27). For scharg (27), the mortality rate for GBS-MFI in very low birthweight infants (<1500) was 75.8%.

9.2.3 Clinical forms associated with mortality

The severity of the clinical picture correlates with the vital prognosis during MFI. Hoover et al (78) reported that mortality was high in neonates who developed **severe respiratory distress**, **severe sepsis** or **meningitis**.

Similarly, the use of mechanical ventilation, high oxygen requirements and the use of vasoactive drugs were significantly associated with a high mortality rate in cases of neonatal infection (200).

Bacterial meningitis can leave long-term sequelae, but is also responsible for high mortality rates (202). Overall mortality in cases of meningitis was 13.7%. It was higher in premature than in term babies, 26.7% versus 9.6%, and in late than in early forms, 16.5% versus 8.2% (202).

Factors associated with a fatal outcome in GBS meningitis described in the literature were prematurity, convulsions before and after the start of treatment, initial shock, coma and assisted ventilation. Biologically, leukopenia, very high protein or very low glucose levels in the initial CSF, a high bacterial concentration in the initial CSF (greater than 106 germs/mL) and unsterilized CSF at the first follow-up LP at H48 were associated with a poor prognosis (116).

In a recent article published in 2020, early neonatal GBS meningitis was associated with 30% mortality (115). Hence the importance of early diagnosis and management.

In the series by Georget-Bouquinet (116), mortality from GBS meningitis was estimated at 14% and immediate complications at 62%, the most frequent being convulsions (45%).

Furthermore, prematurity was considered a risk factor for late meningitis, but not for early neonatal meningitis (116).

9.2.4 Biological signs associated with mortality

With regard to biological risk factors, some studies have reported that thrombocytopenia and leukopenia are factors associated with a high mortality rate (44).

9.3   Risk factors associated with complicated GBS MFIs

Group B streptococcal (GBS) infection was the most common infectious disease in newborns during the first week of life. Morbidity and mortality in GBS-infected newborns were significantly higher than in normal newborns (103,203).

Complicated GBS MFI has been **defined** in some studies as MFI associated with meningitis, severe sepsis and/or septic shock, or severe respiratory distress requiring ventilatory support (114,194).

This rate was lower than that reported in a cohort published in 2021 (36.7%) (114).

The prognosis of GBS MFI depends on several factors. We suspected, as noted in some studies (114), that the occurrence of complicated GBS sepsis and mortality was associated with both neonatal factors and factors related to highly pathogenic GBS strains.

9.3.1 Prematurity

Prematurity is a poor prognostic factor for neonatal infection.

Boyer (70), Trijbels-Smaulders (68) and Joubrel (55) have reported that prematurity is a risk factor for the development of severe sepsis in neonates. Indeed, the greater immaturity of the immune system in the premature infant makes the infection all the more serious on the one hand. On the other hand, the occurrence of early GBS sepsis in the immature neonate was associated with an increased risk of all the complications of prematurity, in particular bronchopulmonary dysplasia and intraventricular hemorrhage or periventricular leukomalacia (23).

9.3.2 Low birth weight

Low birth weight is also one of the factors incriminated in the development of a complicated form during GBS MFI. The latter was more pronounced in babies whose birth weight was below 2,500g.

9.3.3 Association of severe sepsis or septic shock

Severe sepsis remains the most feared complication of MFI.

To date, there is no consensus definition for the diagnosis of neonatal sepsis (106,204). In the various definitions used in the literature, clinical signs, although not specific, must be included in the body of evidence alongside biological and bacteriological signs. In addition, there is no organ dysfunction score for early neonatal infection, whereas well-defined scores are applicable in late neonatal infection to predict the risk of mortality in late neonatal infection (200). The lack of consensus on the diagnosis of neonatal sepsis could be explained by the variability in the sensitivity of clinical and biological criteria. Some studies have found the sensitivity to be 20% for hypothermia or fever, 43% for leukocyte and neutrophil abnormalities and 87% for respiratory distress (106). In fact, fever and thermal instability were difficult criteria to interpret in the setting of severe sepsis, particularly in premature neonates, who are likely to be essentially hypothermic (106). Organ dysfunction factors may include the need for inotropes, intubation in severe respiratory distress, oliguria or coagulopathy (106).

Prognostic factors for neonatal sepsis reported in the literature were inflammatory response, severity and duration of clinical signs (severe respiratory distress with increased oxygen requirement, hemodynamic disturbances such as tachycardia, arterial hypotension) and biological abnormalities mainly neutropenia (106).

9.3.4 Pneumonia Association

In the literature, the appearance of infectious alveolitis in GBS MFI has not been cited as a poor prognostic factor. However, it has been reported that neonatal GBS pneumonia is associated with respiratory distress, most often severe, requiring mechanical ventilation (200).

9.3.5 Biological signs

Recent studies have demonstrated that leukopenia and thrombocytopenia are markers of the severity of MFI (58,95).

Few studies have confirmed the association with anemia (114).

9.3.6 Serotype

According to a systematic review of the literature published in 2020, serotype III strains were the most frequent, accounting for around 50% of early forms. In second place was serotype Ia, detected in MFIs in 22% of cases (205).

According to Lin et al (114), GBS serotype III/ST-17 strains accounted for more than half of all newborns with GBS sepsis and meningitis. In addition, serotype Ib strains were significantly more likely to cause complicated early neonatal infection.

In the study conducted in the Sfax microbiology laboratory in 2020 on early and late GBS neonatal infections (61), the serotype distribution of GBS isolates was similar to that described worldwide. During GBS MFIs, GBS serotype III ST-17 was identified in 17.8% of early GBS MFIs and in 16.7% of cases of early GBS meningitis (61).

9.4 Neurosensory sequelae

The burden of GBS MFI is responsible for medium- and long-term neurodevelopmental disorders (psychomotor retardation, blindness or deafness, cognitive impairment) (206). The risk of neurosensory sequelae during GBS infection was well studied in the literature. The majority of studies included both early and late entities (12,207-210). However, few data have been published concerning the long-term neurological evolution of early neonatal GBS infection.

According to Schuchat (11), 7% of newborns hospitalized for GBS MFI had long-term neurological sequelae. In more recent studies, the authors compared a group of babies with GBS sepsis to a group of babies with no history of GBS MFI, and concluded that the risk of motor impairment was higher (23.5% versus 3.1%) in cases of GBS sepsis (209,210). Furthermore, Nakwa et al (208), in a case-control study, showed that neonates surviving invasive GBS sepsis were 3.5 times more likely than controls to develop neurological disorders at 1 year of age.

These major neurological sequelae were particularly observed in meningeal and complicated forms. According to the literature (199,208,209), 18% to 42% of children with meningitis had permanent neurological sequelae. Nearly two-thirds of babies with complicated GBS sepsis developed at least one neurological complication in the acute or sub-acute phase (114).

According to the literature, bacterial meningitis in newborns, particularly GBS, was a significant cause of neurological sequelae, estimated at between 18 and 42.8% (199,208,209).

Several causal mechanisms have been suggested, including the production of pro-inflammatory cytokines by infectious germs, notably GBS. The neurotoxic effect of these inflammatory cytokines can increase the permeability of the blood-brain barrier in neonates, contributing to brain damage (208,211). Hemodynamic instability and respiratory distress also represent an additional risk of cerebral damage. Hypoxemia and pathological alterations in cerebral blood flow alone can present a risk for neurodevelopment, particularly in premature and hypotrophic newborns. Indeed, premature or low-birth-weight babies with early sepsis had a higher risk of neurological sequelae at 2 years of age (208,211). Prevention of GBS MFI Prophylactic measures are considered in view of the frequency and severity of early neonatal invasive GBS disease and the difficulty of diagnosis. They are aimed at eliminating the germ in the mother and reducing the factors favoring this infection.

9.5 Different strategies for preventing GBS-MFIs

Many industrialized countries, such as the USA, Canada and most of Europe, have adopted a GBS prevention strategy based on universal screening by vaginal and anal swabbing, between 35ème and 37ème SA. Preventive treatment with antibiotic prophylaxis was introduced in the event of positive screening associated with one of the following risk factors: rupture of the water sac lasting more than 18 hours or a maternal temperature $\geq$ 38°C (7,46,201,212). This strategy was responsible for the use of IAP for 26.7% of all pregnant women and for preventing 90% of neonatal infections (68). Other countries, including the UK and the Netherlands, do not actively screen for GBS, but offer IAP to women with prolonged premature rupture of membranes, per-partum fever or GBS UTI during pregnancy (21,213). According to Trijbels-Smeulders (68), with this second strategy based on risk factors, 18% of pregnant women would receive IAP and 69% of neonatal GBS infections would be prevented.

In Sweden, the National Consensus Group, in a study carried out between 2006 and 2011, opted for a risk-factor-based prevention strategy in the face of a high prevalence of GBS carriage and a relatively low rate of GBS-MFI (108). The main finding of this study was a 50% reduction in GBS-MFI in newborns with risk factors for infection (108).

Nevertheless, a meta-analysis published in 2020 comparing the two strategies concluded that protocols based on GBS carriage screening were associated with a lower incidence of GBS MFI compared with protocols based on risk factors (40,74,214). Indeed, positive vaginal swabbing not only enables treatment of carrier women, but also studies antibiotic susceptibility in penicillin-allergic women (215). Similarly, other recent studies (carried out in Europe, America and China) have reported that antibiotic prophylaxis in GBS-positive women could reduce the incidence of GBS MFI by up to 50-80% (23,40,56,216).

In Tunisia, prevention strategies are not yet well defined, and the incidence of neonatal GBS disease remains high.

In fact, GBS screening in pregnant women is not yet routine practice. In a prospective, multicenter study conducted in 2018 in 4 neonatology departments in Tunisia, vaginal swabbing was not performed in only 23.3% of cases, and antibiotic prophylaxis was not complied with in 57.2% of cases (19).

Subsequently, the absence of a GBS screening strategy in our region would partly explain the high frequency of GBS MFI in our series.

Moreover, prevention of GBS infection during pregnancy is complex and influenced by multiple factors. Some studies have shown that preterm delivery, precipitated labor and mothers with negative GBS screening were the main causes of failure of prevention strategies and inadequate IPA (217). For this reason, it is recommended to repeat the PV after 5 weeks if it is negative in women who have not yet given birth (217).

9.6 Intrapartum antibiotic prophylaxis

9.6.1 Benefits of intrapartum antibiotic prophylaxis

The use of AIP has significantly reduced vertical transmission of GBS (9,46) and reduced the incidence of GBS MFIs from 1 to 2 per 1000 NV to 0.5 per 1000 NV (218).

In a meta-analysis published in 2012, studies reporting the use of IPA found a lower incidence of GBS MFI (0.23 per 1000 NV) compared with studies in which women had not used prophylaxis (0.75 per 1000 NV) (25).

Nevertheless, the majority of low-income countries do not have a prevention policy, and implementation of recommendations is difficult, which explains the increase in the incidence of MFIs (7,30).

In a multi-center Tunisian study, Badri et al (19) demonstrated that AIP significantly reduced the length of hospital stay for neonates with suspected MFI (p=0.041).

9.6.2 Indications for intrapartum antibiotic prophylaxis

According to the 2017 SFN (194) and 2010 CDC (46) recommendations, intrapartum antibiotic prophylaxis is indicated in cases of:

- Maternal fever > 38°C intrapartum, isolated or associated with signs of chorioamniotitis, regardless of the status of the vaginal swab.

- Known maternal GBS colonization during current pregnancy (positive vaginal swab or GBS bacteriuria).

- A history of neonatal GBS infection in a previous pregnancy.

- In case of unknown status of vaginal swab, AIP is administered in case of RPM > 12 hours (for SFN) 18 hours (for CDC) or in case of spontaneous and unexplained prematurity < 37 SA.

Thus, any woman who presents without a vaginal swab is assumed to have a GBS carrier and should receive an IAP if she has any other risk factor for MFI (PMR, threat of premature delivery, fever or signs of chorioamniotitis). This is the most frequent situation for women who come to give birth in our country (23.3% of women alone have a PV), particularly in our region of Sfax.

9.6.3 Molecules used for intrapartum antibiotic prophylaxis

Antibiotic prophylaxis reduces maternal vaginal colonization peri-partum. Antibiotics can reach bactericidal levels in fetal blood within minutes of intrapartum administration, and high neonatal blood concentrations persist for hours after birth (108).

Penicillin G at an initial dose of 5 million units, followed by 3 million units every 4 hours, and Ampicillin at an initial dose of 2g, followed by 1g every 4 hours, are the molecules of choice for AIP (219). In fact, these molecules have a narrower spectrum of antimicrobial activity than the 3ème generation cephalosporins, thereby limiting the potential selection of resistant germs. In addition, their pharmacokinetics are well adapted (220,221).

The CDC recommends Cefazolin at an initial dose of 2g, then 1g every 8 hours in cases of penicillin allergy with a low risk of anaphylaxis (46). Erythromycin is no longer recommended for MFI prophylaxis due to high resistance rates. In the case of life-threatening penicillin allergy (history of anaphylaxis, rash, angioedema, respiratory symptoms), Clindamycin at a dose of 900mg every 8 hours is the antibiotic prophylaxis of choice, after sensitivity testing. If Clindamycin is of unknown or low sensitivity, vancomycin is indicated as antibiotic prophylaxis (46,219). The recommended dose is 20mg/kg every 8 hours, with a maximum dose of 2g (219).

Good antibiotic prophylaxis consists of at least one dose of one of the above-mentioned molecules, administered **intravenously** at least **four hours** before birth. Although a shorter duration between antibiotic prophylaxis and delivery is less effective, 2 hours of antibiotic exposure has been shown to reduce the risk of neonatal sepsis (222). Furthermore, Barbier et al (223), in their prospective cohort study, concluded that fetuses exposed to less than 4 hours of prophylaxis had higher penicillin G levels than those exposed to more than 4 hours (p = 0.003).

9.6.4 Adverse effects of intrapartum antibiotic prophylaxis

This antibiotic prophylaxis exposes the woman and her newborn to antibiotics, whereas only 1-2% of newborns are reported to have developed invasive GBS disease (46). This increase in perinatal antibiotic prophylaxis is associated with a change in the pathogens responsible for sepsis in premature and very-low-birth-weight babies. At the same time, concerns have arisen about a possible increase in the incidence of neonatal gram-negative bacillus (GNB) infections, notably due to resistant strains of E. coli (218,224,225). Moreover, this antibiotic prophylaxis does not reduce the incidence of late GBS infections (218,226).

In addition, researchers have shown that antibiotic use in neonates is associated with increased risk of health problems later in childhood (food allergies, asthma, inflammatory bowel disease and childhood obesity) (137). It can be concluded that routine antibiotic prophylaxis does not appear to be beneficial in reducing neonatal infection or mortality compared with close monitoring and selective antibiotics.

9.7   Rapid tests for the detection of GBS colonization

The development of new, more reliable and less expensive rapid diagnostic tests for GBS may change the practice of systematic maternal screening. Instead of taking a sample in the 3rd trimester, it will then be possible to carry out a test on admission to the delivery room, with results available in just a few minutes. This would enable us to offer antibiotic prophylaxis only to parturients who actually carry GBS during labor (121). This type of test should be easily integrated into laboratory routines and available at any time. However, they are not sufficiently sensitive to detect mild colonization.

They are not suitable to replace prenatal screening by culture. A positive result from a rapid test performed at the time of labor would be considered as positive GBS status for the pregnant woman, but a negative result has no significance (40).

At present, these rapid tests for GBS antigen detection on vaginal smears are not available in Tunisia.

More recently, **a real-time PCR detection test** with good sensitivity (100%) and specificity (97%) has become available in early labor (40). This test is proving very promising for the rapid and appropriate detection of GBS on vaginal smears, and offers the advantage of establishing GBS colonization status on admission of parturients who have not had prenatal follow-up.

Nevertheless, rapid PCR testing is more expensive than swab culture. What's more, it can take up to 2 hours to obtain a result. This is important, as the maximum benefit of AIP is only achieved when it is administered for at least two (and preferably four) hours before birth. An additional disadvantage of PCR-based intrapartum tests is that they cannot provide information about GBS resistance to the antibiotics used for AIP (40). Randomized trials of prophylaxis based on prenatal culture and PCR testing in early labor are underway.

We have shown that preventive measures are not always available. All the more so as AIP may be more difficult to apply due to late presentation to health facilities. Maternal vaccination is therefore an alternative strategy.

9.8 Vaccination against group B Streptococcus

As early as the 1930s, Rebbeca Lancefield demonstrated the protective immunity of polyclonal antibodies directed against the GBS capsule. Based on the relationship between maternal immunoglobulin levels and the risk of neonatal infection, capsule-directed vaccines are still being developed today. Nevertheless, the low level of cross-protection between the different serotypes has highlighted the importance of implementing a multi-valent vaccine (205).

A pentavalent conjugate vaccine (Ia/Ib/II/III/V) covers almost all pathogenic neonatal serotypes worldwide (96%) (9). But it cannot cover serotype IV, which recently emerged in the United States. This is why more recent studies speak of hexavalent vaccines (Ia/Ib/II/III/IV/V) which have the potential to prevent up to 93% of maternal colonizations worldwide, 99% of invasive neonatal infections and 99% of stillbirths (205).

ST-17 strains were responsible for the majority of neonatal meningitis cases. Although the majority of ST-17 isolates belonged to serotype III, the invasiveness of ST-17 was independent of capsular serotype (227). Coverage of ST-17 strains is necessary in the GBS vaccine.

Reducing maternal infections, perinatal morbidity and mortality, and late sequelae of neonatal GBS infections are the major health and economic impacts of vaccines. Maternal GBS vaccines could overcome the disadvantages of antibiotic prophylaxis, reducing antibiotic use and effects on the overall microbiome of mother and neonate, and help reduce the development of antibiotic resistance (228).

Thus, GBS vaccines are the most effective and longest-lasting preventive strategy. To date, however, there is no licensed vaccine available in routine practice (40,227).

In Tunisia, the problem is even more acute: on the one hand, the practice of PV and AIP is still limited, and on the other, the absence of microbiology laboratories in certain regions increases the risk of GBS MFIs. For this reason, we have proposed a GBS prevention protocol adapted to our local conditions, with the aim of reducing the burden of this serious pathology, as well as a protocol for the management of term babies ≥ 34SA born to GBS-colonized mothers.

Table V: Proposed GBS MFI prevention protocol

Systematic screening for maternal GBS carriage:

- Take a vaginal swab (PV) and rectal swab at the end of pregnancy, between **36 and 38** weeks' gestation.

- For women who have not been screened at the end of pregnancy, we suggest performing a PV or rapid PCR test per-partum on admission.

- - The PV must be repeated after 5 weeks of a GBS-negative PV if the mother has not yet given birth.

Specify on the request that you are looking for GBS, and if you are allergic to penicillin, ask for an antibiotic susceptibility test.

Indications for antibiotic prophylaxis (API) in the presence of at least one of the following risk factors:

- PV positive for GBS.

- History of neonatal GBS infection in a previous pregnancy

- GBS bacteriuria during pregnancy at any term

- Intrapartum temperature $\geq 38°C$ or signs of chorioamniotitis

- Threat of premature and unexplained delivery $< 37SA$

- Rupture of membranes ≥ 12 hours

Start antibiotic prophylaxis as early as possible in labor, as it is most effective after the 2eme injection.

Recommended intrapartum antibiotic prophylaxis regimens

- **Penicillin G** (5 MU then 2.5 MU / 4 hours) or **amoxicillin** (2g then 1g/4 hours) until delivery

In case of allergy to penicillin and according to the antibiotic susceptibility test

If exposed to a low risk of anaphylaxis: **Cefazolin** (2g then 1g /8 hours) until delivery.

If exposed to a high risk of anaphylaxis: **Clindamycin** (900mg /8 hours) or
- **Vancomycin** (1g /12 hours), until delivery

Intravenous

At **least 4 hours before birth**

PV: vaginal swab; PCR: polymerase chain reaction; SGB: Streptococcus B; AIP: intrapartum antibiotic prophylaxis; SA: weeks of amenorrhea.

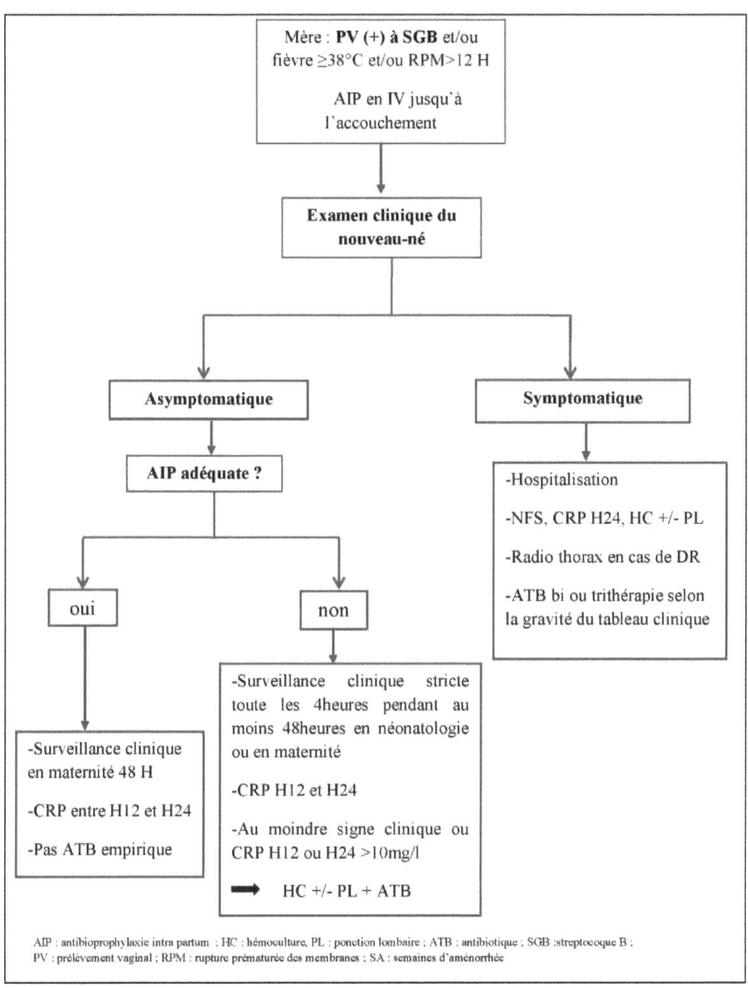

Figure 2: Management of the newborn of a mother colonized with GBS and whose term ≥34 SA

Conclusion

Maternal-fetal infection (MFI) with Group B Streptococcus (GBS) continues to be a constant preoccupation for pediatricians and obstetricians. On the one hand, it remains a serious pathology that can be life-threatening for newborn babies. On the other hand, it poses a problem of diagnosis and management, due to the lack of specificity of clinical signs and the delay in bacteriological diagnosis.

GBS is particularly interesting to study, since most early neonatal GBS infections can be prevented by the use of specific preventive measures based on screening for maternal GBS carriage and intrapartum antibiotic prophylaxis (IPP) for colonized women.

However, its incidence remains high in some countries, particularly in Africa.

Prevention therefore requires ongoing collaboration between obstetricians, neontologists, microbiologists and biologists.

It is for this reason that we have proposed a GBS prevention protocol adapted to our local conditions, with the aim of reducing the burden of this serious pathology.

This protocol is based on antibiotic prophylaxis for women with a history of GBS FMD, GBS bacteriuria, premature delivery, maternal fever and/or chorioamniotitis or premature rupture of membranes > 12 hours, and women colonized with GBS late in pregnancy. Routine screening for GBS in all pregnant women is therefore necessary between 34 and 38 weeks' gestation.

Thereafter, clinical monitoring is essential for all neonates at high risk of infection. In fact, clinical monitoring by competent neonatal staff during the stay in the maternity ward or neonatal unit is imperative for the early recognition of clinical signs of MFI and the timely administration of appropriate antibiotic treatment.

Thanks to these preventive measures, the incidence of early neonatal GBS infection could be reduced.

Vaccinating mothers against GBS could be a more effective prevention strategy for both early and late neonatal infection.

Bibliographies

1. Puopolo KM, Benitz WE, Zaoutis TE, COMMITTEE ON FETUS AND NEWBORN, COMMITTEE ON INFECTIOUS DISEASES, Cummings J, et al. Management of Neonates Born at ≥35 0/7 Weeks' Gestation With Suspected or Proven Early-Onset Bacterial Sepsis. Pediatrics. 1 Dec 2018;142(6).

2. Russell NJ, Seale AC, O'Driscoll M, O'Sullivan C, Bianchi-Jassir F, Gonzalez-Guarin J, et al. Maternal Colonization With Group B Streptococcus and Serotype Distribution Worldwide: Systematic Review and Meta-analyses. Clin Infect Dis. 15 Nov 2017;65(Suppl 2):S100-11.

3. Hall J, Adams NH, Bartlett L, Seale AC, Lamagni T, Bianchi-Jassir F, et al. Maternal Disease With Group B Streptococcus and Serotype Distribution Worldwide: Systematic Review and Meta-analyses. Clin Infect Dis. 6 Nov 2017;65(suppl_2):S112-24.

4. Seale AC, Bianchi-Jassir F, Russell NJ, Kohli-Lynch M, Tann CJ, Hall J, et al. Estimates of the Burden of Group B Streptococcal Disease Worldwide for Pregnant Women, Stillbirths, and Children. Clin Infect Dis. Nov 6, 2017;65(suppl_2):S200-19.

5. Seale AC, Blencowe H, Bianchi-Jassir F, Embleton N, Bassat Q, Ordi J, et al. Stillbirth With Group B Streptococcus Disease Worldwide: Systematic Review and Metaanalyses. Clin Infect Dis. 6 Nov 2017;65(suppl_2):S125-32.

6. Poyart C, Tazi A, Réglier-Poupet H, Billoët A, Tavares N, Raymond J, et al. Multiplex PCR Assay for Rapid and Accurate Capsular Typing of Group B Streptococci. Journal of Clinical Microbiology. June 2007;45(6):1985.

7. Le Doare K, O'Driscoll M, Turner K, Seedat F, Russell NJ, Seale AC, et al. Intrapartum Antibiotic Chemoprophylaxis Policies for the Prevention of Group B Streptococcal Disease Worldwide: Systematic Review. Clin Infect Dis. Nov 6, 2017;65(suppl_2):S143-51.

8. Schrag SJ, Verani JR. Intrapartum antibiotic prophylaxis for the prevention of perinatal group B streptococcal disease: experience in the United States and implications for a potential group B streptococcal vaccine. Vaccine. August 28, 2013;31 Suppl 4:D20-26.

9. Madrid L, Seale AC, Kohli-Lynch M, Edmond KM, Lawn JE, Heath PT, et al. Infant Group B Streptococcal Disease Incidence and Serotypes Worldwide: Systematic Review and Meta-analyses. Clin Infect Dis. Nov 6, 2017;65(suppl_2):S160-72.

10. WHO Urges Vaccine Against Bacteria Killing 150,000 Babies Each Year

11. Schuchat A. Epidemiology of Group B Streptococcal Disease in the United States: Shifting Paradigms. Clin Microbiol Rev. Jul 1998;11(3):497-513.

12. Kohli-Lynch M, Russell NJ, Seale AC, Dangor Z, Tann CJ, Baker CJ, et al. Neurodevelopmental Impairment in Children After Group B Streptococcal Disease Worldwide: Systematic Review and Meta-analyses. Clin Infect Dis. 15 Nov 2017;65(Suppl 2):S190-9.

13. Ben Hamida Nouaili E, Abidi K, Chaouachi S, Marrakchi Z. Epidemiology of maternal- fetal group B streptococcal infections. Med Mal Infect. March 2011;41(3):123-5.

14. Ben Hamida Nouaili E, Harouni M, Chaouachi S, Sfar R, Marrakchi Z. Early-onset neonatal bacterial infections: a retrospective series of 144 cases. Tunis Med. Feb 2008;86(2):136-9.

15. Bahloul M, al. L'infection materno-foetale à Streptocoque du groupe B: à propos de 75 cas [thèse]. [Sfax]: Faculté de médecine Sfax; 2012.

16. Dermer P, Lee C, Eggert J, Few B. A history of neonatal group B streptococcus with its related morbidity and mortality rates in the United States. J Pediatr Nurs. Oct 2004;19(5):357-63.

17. Gras-Le Guen C, Foix-L'Hélias L, Boileau P. Early neonatal bacterial infection (EBNI): what algorithm for management in 2017? Archives de Pédiatrie. Dec 1, 2017;24:S14-7.

18. ANES E. Diagnosis et traitement curatif de l'infection bactérienne précoce du nouveau- né: Septembre 2002, Service des recommandations et références professionnelles. EMConsulte.

19. Badri MA, al. Nouveau protocole devant une suspicion d'infection néonatale précoce bactérienne asymptomatique [thèse]. [Tunisia]: Faculté de médecine Sfax; 2020.

20. Phares CR, Lynfield R, Farley MM, Mohle-Boetani J, Harrison LH, Petit S, et al. Epidemiology of invasive group B streptococcal disease in the United States, 1999-2005. JAMA. May 7, 2008;299(17):2056-65.

21. Bekker V, Bijlsma MW, van de Beek D, Kuijpers TW, van der Ende A. Incidence of invasive group B streptococcal disease and pathogen genotype distribution in newborn babies in the Netherlands over 25 years: a nationwide surveillance study. Lancet Infect Dis. nov 2014;14(11):1083-9.

22. Six A, Joubrel C, Tazi A, Poyart C. Maternal-fetal infections with Streptococcus agalactiae. La Presse Médicale. June 1, 2014;43(6, Part 1):706-14.

23. Stoll BJ, Hansen NI, Sánchez PJ, Faix RG, Poindexter BB, Van Meurs KP, et al. Early Onset Neonatal Sepsis: The Burden of Group B Streptococcal and E. coli Disease Continues. Pediatrics. May 2011;127(5):817-26.

24. Carbonell-Estrany X, Figueras-Aloy J, Salcedo-Abizanda S, de la Rosa-Fraile M, Castrillo Study Group. Probable early-onset group B streptococcal

neonatal sepsis: a serious clinical condition related to intrauterine infection. Arch Dis Child Fetal Neonatal Ed. March 2008;93(2):F85-89.

25. Nanduri SA, Petit S, Smelser C, Apostol M, Alden NB, Harrison LH, et al. Epidemiology of Invasive Early-Onset and Late-Onset Group B Streptococcal Disease in the United States, 2006 to 2015: Multistate Laboratory and Population-Based Surveillance. JAMA Pediatr. March 1, 2019;173(3):224-33.

26. Schrag SJ, Schuchat A. Easing the Burden: Characterizing the Disease Burden of Neonatal Group B Streptococcal Disease to Motivate Prevention. Clinical Infectious Diseases. May 1, 2004;38(9):1209-11.

27. Schrag SJ, Farley MM, Petit S, Reingold A, Weston EJ, Pondo T, et al. Epidemiology of Invasive Early-Onset Neonatal Sepsis, 2005 to 2014. Pediatrics. dec 2016;138(6):e20162013.

28. Kuhn P, Dheu C, Bolender C, Chognot D, Keller L, Demil H, et al. Incidence and distribution of pathogens in early-onset neonatal sepsis in the era of antenatal antibiotics. Paediatr Perinat Epidemiol. Sept 2010;24(5):479-87.

29. Cutland CL, Schrag SJ, Thigpen MC, Velaphi SC, Wadula J, Adrian PV, et al. Increased risk for group B Streptococcus sepsis in young infants exposed to HIV, Soweto, South Africa, 2004-2008(1). Emerg Infect Dis. Apr 2015;21(4):638-45.

30. Verani JR, Schrag SJ. Group B streptococcal disease in infants: progress in prevention and continued challenges. Clin Perinatol. June 2010;37(2):375-92.

31. Berardi A, Lugli L, Baronciani D, Creti R, Rossi K, Ciccia M, et al. Group B streptococcal infections in a northern region of Italy. Pediatrics. Sept 2007;120(3):e487-493.

32. Tiskumara R, Fakharee SH, Liu CQ, Nuntnarumit P, Lui KM, Hammoud M, et al. Neonatal infections in Asia. Arch Dis Child Fetal Neonatal Ed. March 2009;94(2):F144-148.

33. Gray KJ, Bennett SL, French N, Phiri AJ, Graham SM. Invasive Group B Streptococcal Infection in Infants, Malawi. Emerg Infect Dis. Feb 2007;13(2):223-9.

34. Sinha A, Russell LB, Tomczyk S, Verani JR, Schrag SJ, Berkley JA, et al. Disease Burden of Group B Streptococcus Among Infants in Sub-Saharan Africa: A Systematic Literature Review and Meta-analysis. Pediatr Infect Dis J. Sep 1, 2016;35(9):933-42.

35. Jennifer R, verani, Lesley M, Stephanie J. Prevention of Perinatal Group B Streptococcal Disease. CDC 2010. Nov 19, 2010;59(RR-10):1-32.

36. Nicolay N, Thiolet J-M, Talon D, Poujol I, Bernet C, Carbonne A, et al. Reporting of nosocomial Pseudomonas aeruginosa infections, France, August 2001 - June 2006. :20.

37. Ben Mlik L, al. L'infection materno-foetale à Streptocoque de groupe B: Apropos de 52 observations [Thèse]. [Tunisia]: Faculté de médecine Tunis; 2005.

38. Fekih I. Profile of early maternal-fetal bacterial infections. ThD med [thesis]. [Mahdia, Tunisia]: Faculté de médecine sfax; 2013.

39. Berardi A, Lugli L, Baronciani D, Rossi C, Ciccia M, Creti R, et al. Group B Streptococcus early-onset disease in Emilia-romagna: review after introduction of a screening-based approach. Pediatr Infect Dis J. Feb 2010;29(2):115-21.

40. Steer PJ, Russell AB, Kochhar S, Cox P, Plumb J, Gopal Rao G. Group B streptococcal disease in the mother and newborn-A review. Eur J Obstet Gynecol Reprod Biol. Sept 2020;252:526-33.

41. Baeringsdottir B, Erlendsdottir H, Bjornsdottir ES, Martins ER, Ramirez M, Haraldsson A, et al. Group B streptococcal infections in infants in Iceland: clinical and microbiological factors. Journal of Medical Microbiology;70(9):001426.

42. Morcel K, Lavoué V, Vandenbrouke L, Damaj L, Lassel L, Issly H, et al. Maternal-fetal bacterial infection (excluding listeriosis) - EM consulte.

43. Doran KS, Nizet V. Molecular pathogenesis of neonatal group B streptococcal infection: no longer in its infancy. Molecular Microbiology. 2004;54(1):23-31.

44. Heath PT, Jardine LA. Neonatal infections: group B streptococcus. BMJ Clin Evid. 27 Sep 2010;2010:0323.

45. Parente V, Clark RH, Ku L, Fennell C, Johnson M, Morris E, et al. Risk factors for group B streptococcal disease in neonates of mothers with negative antenatal testing. J Perinatol. 2017;37(2):157-61.

46. Verani JR, McGee L, Schrag SJ, Division of Bacterial Diseases, National Center for Immunization and Respiratory Diseases, Centers for Disease Control and Prevention (CDC). Prevention of perinatal group B streptococcal disease--revised guidelines from CDC, 2010. MMWR Recomm Rep. Nov 19, 2010;59(RR-10):1-36.

47. Alemayehu A, Alemayehu M, Arba A, Abebe H, Goa A, Paulos K, et al. Predictors of Neonatal Sepsis in Hospitals at Wolaita Sodo Town, Southern Ethiopia: InstitutionBased Unmatched Case-Control Study, 2019. Int J Pediatr. 2020;2020:3709672.

48. Jauréguy F, Carton M, Teboul J, Butel M-J, Panel P, Ghnassia J-C, et al. Risk factors and screening strategy for group B streptococcal colonization in pregnant women: Results of a prospective study. Journal of Gynecology, Obstetrics and Reproductive Biology. May 1, 2003;32:132-8.

49. Rao GG, Nartey G, McAree T, O'Reilly A, Hiles S, Lee T, et al. Outcome of a screening programme for the prevention of neonatal invasive early-onset group B Streptococcus infection in a UK maternity unit: An observational

study. BMJ Open. 1 Apr 2017;7(4):e014634.

50. Santhanam S, Arun S, Rebekah G, Ponmudi NJ, Chandran J, Jose R, et al. Perinatal Risk Factors for Neonatal Early-onset Group B Streptococcal Sepsis after Initiation of Risk-based Maternal Intrapartum Antibiotic Prophylaxis-A Case Control Study. J Trop Pediatr. August 1, 2018;64(4):312-6.

51. Yancey MK, Duff P, Kubilis P, Clark P, Frentzen BH. Risk factors for neonatal sepsis. Obstetrics & Gynecology. Feb 1, 1996;87(2):188-94.

52. Adair CE, Kowalsky L, Quon H, Ma D, Stoffman J, McGeer A, et al. Risk factors for early-onset group B streptococcal disease in neonates: a population-based case-control study. CMAJ. August 5, 2003;169(3):198-203.

53. Shane AL, Stoll BJ. Neonatal sepsis: progress toward improved outcomes. J Infect. Jan 2014;68 Suppl 1:S24-32.

54. Lyytikainen O, Nuorti JP, Halmesmaki E, Carlson P, Uotila J, Vuento R, et al. Invasive group B streptococcal infections in Finland: a population-based study. Emerg Infect Dis. Apr 2003;9(4):469-73.

55. Joubrel C, Tazi A, Six A, Dmytruk N, Touak G, Bidet P, et al. Group B streptococcus neonatal invasive infections, France 2007-2012. Clin Microbiol Infect. oct 2015;21(10):910-6.

56. Puopolo KM, Draper D, Wi S, Newman TB, Zupancic J, Lieberman E, et al. Estimating the probability of neonatal early-onset infection on the basis of maternal risk factors. Pediatrics. nov 2011;128(5):e1155-1163.

57. Cho C-Y, Tang Y-H, Chen Y-H, Wang S-Y, Yang Y-H, Wang T-H, et al. Group B Streptococcal infection in neonates and colonization in pregnant women: An epidemiological retrospective analysis. J Microbiol Immunol Infect. Apr 2019;52(2):265-72.

58. Al-Kadri HM, Bamuhair SS, Johani SMA, Al-Buriki NA, Tamim HM. Maternal and neonatal risk factors for early-onset group B streptococcal disease: a case control study. Int J Womens Health. 2013;5:729-35.

59. Chan GJ, Lee ACC, Baqui AH, Tan J, Black RE. Prevalence of early-onset neonatal infection among newborns of mothers with bacterial infection or colonization: a systematic review and meta-analysis. BMC Infect Dis. March 7, 2015;15:118.

60. H H. Prevalence, Antimicrobial Susceptibility and Macrolide Molecular Study in Vaginal Group B Streptococcus: A Five-Year Study among Pregnant Women Attending Antenatal Clinics in a Tertiary Care Hospital in Tunisia. Research and Reviews of Infectious Diseases. 26 Nov 2020;3(2).

61. Kharrat R, al. Group B Streptococcus and perinatality: epidemiological study, serotype distribution and antibiotic susceptibility [thesis]. [Tunisia]: Faculté de médecine Sfax; 2021.

62. Puopolo KM, Madoff LC, Eichenwald EC. Early-onset group B streptococcal disease in the era of maternal screening. Pediatrics. May 2005;115(5):1240-6.

63. Polin RA, Committee on Fetus and Newborn. Management of neonates with suspected or proven early-onset bacterial sepsis. Pediatrics. May 2012;129(5):1006-15.

64. Van Dyke MK, Phares CR, Lynfield R, Thomas AR, Arnold KE, Craig AS, et al. Evaluation of Universal Antenatal Screening for Group B Streptococcus. New England Journal of Medicine. June 18, 2009;360(25):2626-36.

65. Zhu Y, Gao L, Huang Z-L, Wu J-Y, Ni Y, Wang Y-J, et al. Current status of group B Streptococcus infection in neonates: a multicenter prospective study. Zhongguo Dang Dai Er Ke Za Zhi. 15 Sep 2021;23(9):889-95.

66. Konrad G, Katz A. Epidemiology of early-onset neonatal group B streptococcal infection: implications for screening. Can Fam Physician. June 2007;53(6):1055, 2001:e.1-6, 1054.

67. Accoceberry M, Carbonnier M, Boeuf B, Ughetto S, Sapin V, Vendittelli F, et al. Neonatal morbidity after expectant attitude followed by systematic birth at 34 weeks of amenorrhea in situation of premature rupture of membranes. Gynecologie Obstetrique & Fertilite - GYNECOL OBSTET FERTIL. 1 sept 2005;33:577-81.

68. Trijbels-Smeulders M, de Jonge GA, Jong PCMP, Gerards LJ, Adriaanse AH, van Lingen RA, et al. Epidemiology of neonatal group B streptococcal disease in the Netherlands before and after introduction of guidelines for prevention. Arch Dis Child Fetal Neonatal Ed. Jul 2007;92(4):F271-6.

69. G/eyesus T, Moges F, Eshetie S, Yeshitela B, Abate E. Bacterial etiologic agents causing neonatal sepsis and associated risk factors in Gondar, Northwest Ethiopia. BMC Pediatr. June 6, 2017;17:137.

70. Boyer KM, Gotoff SP. Prevention of early-onset neonatal group B streptococcal disease with selective intrapartum chemoprophylaxis. N Engl J Med. June 26, 1986;314(26):1665-9.

71. Avila C, Willins JL, Jackson M, Mathai J, Jabsky M, Kong A, et al. Usefulness of two clinical chorioamnionitis definitions in predicting neonatal infectious outcomes: a systematic review. Am J Perinatol. sept 2015;32(11):1001-9.

72. Astruc D, Zores C, Dillenseger L, Scheib C, Kuhn P. [Practical management of neonatal sepsis risk in term or near-term infants]. Arch Pediatr. Sept 2014;21(9):1041-8.

73. Lin FY, Brenner RA, Johnson YR, Azimi PH, Philips JB, Regan JA, et al. The effectiveness of risk-based intrapartum chemoprophylaxis for the prevention of early-onset neonatal group B streptococcal disease. Am J Obstet Gynecol.

May 2001;184(6):1204-10.

74. Schrag SJ, Zell ER, Lynfield R, Roome A, Arnold KE, Craig AS, et al. A population-based comparison of strategies to prevent early-onset group B streptococcal disease in neonates. N Engl J Med. 25 Jul 2002;347(4):233-9.

75. Todorova-Christova M, Vacheva R, Decheva A, Nikolov A, Slancheva B, Stoichkova D, et al. A study on early-onset neonatal group B streptococcal infection, Bulgaria, 20072011. Arch Pediatr. Sept 2014;21(9):953-60.

76. Shrestha RK, Rai SK, Khanal LK, Manda PK. Bacteriological study of neonatal sepsis and antibiotic susceptibility pattern of isolates in Kathmandu, Nepal. Nepal Med Coll J. March 2013;15(1):71-3.

77. Leineweber B, Grote V, Schaad UB, Heininger U. Transplacentally acquired immunoglobulin G antibodies against measles, mumps, rubella and varicella-zoster virus in preterm and full term newborns. Pediatr Infect Dis J. Apr 2004;23(4):361-3.

78. Hoover LE. Group B Streptococcus Disease: AAP Updates Guidelines for the Management of At-Risk Infants. Am Fam Physician. 15 2020;101(6):378-80.

79. Pass MA, Khare S, Dillon HC. Twin pregnancies: incidence of group B streptococcal colonization and disease. J Pediatr. Oct 1980;97(4):635-7.

80. Doran KS, Benoit VM, Gertz RE, Beall B, Nizet V. Late-Onset Group B Streptococcal Infection in Identical Twins: Insight to Disease Pathogenesis. J Perinatol. June 2002;22(4):326-30.

81. Sgro M, Kobylianskii A, Yudin MH, Tran D, Diamandakos J, Sgro J, et al. Populationbased study of early-onset neonatal sepsis in Canada. Paediatr Child Health. May 2019;24(2):e66-73.

82. Russell NJ, Seale AC, O'Sullivan C, Le Doare K, Heath PT, Lawn JE, et al. Risk of Early-Onset Neonatal Group B Streptococcal Disease With Maternal Colonization Worldwide: Systematic Review and Meta-analyses. Clin Infect Dis. Nov 6, 2017;65(suppl_2):S152-9.

83. Stoll BJ, Hansen N, Fanaroff AA, Wright LL, Carlo WA, Ehrenkranz RA, et al. Changes in pathogens causing early-onset sepsis in very-low-birth-weight infants. N Engl J Med. July 25 2002;347(4):240-7.

84. Weston EJ, Pondo T, Lewis MM, Martell-Cleary P, Morin C, Jewell B, et al. The burden of invasive early-onset neonatal sepsis in the United States, 2005-2008. Pediatr Infect Dis J. Nov 2011;30(11):937-41.

85. Fluegge K, Siedler A, Heinrich B, Schulte-Moenting J, Moennig M-J, Bartels DB, et al. Incidence and clinical presentation of invasive neonatal group B streptococcal infections in Germany. Pediatrics. June 2006;117(6):e1139-1145.

86. Ben Zayed C. Early maternal-fetal infections: epidemiological, clinical, bacteriological and therapeutic aspects [Thesis]. Faculty of Medicine Tunis; 2016.

87. Pandit BR, Vyas A. Clinical Symptoms, Pathogen Spectrum, Risk factors and Antibiogram of Suspected Neonatal Sepsis cases in Tertiary Care Hospital of Southern Part of Nepal: A Descriptive Cross-sectional Study. JNMA J Nepal Med Assoc. Dec 2020;58(232):976-82.

88. Boyer KM, Gadzala CA, Kelly PD, Burd LI, Gotoff SP. Selective intrapartum chemoprophylaxis of neonatal group B streptococcal early-onset disease. II. Predictive value of prenatal cultures. J Infect Dis. Nov 1983;148(5):802-9.

89. Heath PT, Jardine LA. Neonatal infections: group B streptococcus. BMJ Clin Evid. 28 Feb 2014;2014:0323.

90. Benitz WE, Gould JB, Druzin ML. Risk factors for early-onset group B streptococcal sepsis: estimation of odds ratios by critical literature review. Pediatrics. June 1999;103(6):e77.

91. Jackson GL, Engle WD, Sendelbach DM, Vedro DA, Josey S, Vinson J, et al. Are complete blood cell counts useful in the evaluation of asymptomatic neonates exposed to suspected chorioamnionitis? Pediatrics. May 2004;113(5):1173-80.

92. Wang ME, Patel AB, Hansen NI, Arlington L, Prakash A, Hibberd PL. Risk factors for possible serious bacterial infection in a rural cohort of young infants in central India. BMC Public Health. 19 Oct 2016;16(1):1097.

93. Szymusik I, Kosinska-Kaczyinska K, Pietrzak B, Wielgos M. [Do we need a different approach to GBS screening?]. Ginekol Pol. June 2014;85(6):456-60.

94. Zaleznik DF, Rench MA, Hillier S, Krohn MA, Platt R, Lee M-LT, et al. Invasive Disease Due to Group B Streptococcus in Pregnant Women and Neonates from Diverse Population Groups. Clinical Infectious Diseases. Feb 2000;30(2):276-81.

95. Bromberger P, Lawrence JM, Braun D, Saunders B, Contreras R, Petitti DB. The Influence of Intrapartum Antibiotics on the Clinical Spectrum of Early-Onset Group B Streptococcal Infection in Term Infants. Pediatrics. August 1, 2000;106(2):244-50.

96. Shah BA, Padbury JF. Neonatal sepsis. Virulence. 1 Jan 2014;5(1):170-8.

97. Lannering B, Larsson LE, Rojas J, Stahlman MT. Early onset group B streptococcal disease. Seven year experience and clinical scoring system. Acta Paediatr Scand. July 1983;72(4):597-602.

98. Aujard Y. 4 - Manifestations cliniques des infections néonatales: Clinical manifestations of neonatal infections. In: Aujard Y, editor. Infections néonatales. Paris: Elsevier Masson; 2015. p. 27-34.

99. Li X, Ding X, Shi P, Zhu Y, Huang Y, Li Q, et al. Clinical features and antimicrobial susceptibility profiles of culture-proven neonatal sepsis in a tertiary children's hospital, 2013 to 2017. Medicine (Baltimore). march 2019;98(12):e14686.

100. Jain NK, Jain VM, Maheshwari S. Clinical profile of neonatal sepsis. Kathmandu Univ Med J (KUMJ). June 2003;1(2):117-20.

101. Andersen J, Christensen R, Hertel J. Clinical features and epidemiology of septicaemia and meningitis in neonates due to Streptococcus agalactiae in Copenhagen County, Denmark: a 10-year survey from 1992 to 2001. Acta Paediatr. Oct 2004;93(10):1334-9.

102. de Gier B, van Kassel MN, Sanders EAM, van de Beek D, Hahné SJM, van der Ende A, et al. Disease burden of neonatal invasive Group B Streptococcus infection in the Netherlands. PLoS ONE. 2019;14(5):e0216749.

103. Carlough MC, Crowell K, Richard N. Clinical inquiries. How should we manage infants at risk for group B streptococcal disease? J Fam Pract. May 2003;52(5):406, 408-9.

104. Ji W, Liu H, Madhi SA, Cunnington M, Zhang Z, Dangor Z, et al. Clinical and Molecular Epidemiology of Invasive Group B Streptococcus Disease among Infants, China. Emerg Infect Dis. nov 2019;25(11):2021-30.

105. Wynn JL, Polin RA. Progress in the management of neonatal sepsis: the importance of a consensus definition. Pediatr Res. Jan 2018;83(1-1):13-5.

106. Wynn JL, Wong HR, Shanley TP, Bizzarro MJ, Saiman L, Polin RA. Time for a Neonatal-Specific Consensus Definition for Sepsis. Pediatric Critical Care Medicine. july 2014;15(6):523-8.

107. National Collaborating Centre for Women's and Children's Health (UK). Antibiotics for Early-Onset Neonatal Infection: Antibiotics for the Prevention and Treatment of Early- Onset Neonatal Infection. London: RCOG Press; 2012. (National Institute for Health and Clinical Excellence: Guidance).

108. Hâkansson S, Lilja M, Jacobsson B, Kallén K. Reduced incidence of neonatal early-onset group B streptococcal infection after promulgation of guidelines for risk-based intrapartum antibiotic prophylaxis in Sweden: analysis of a national population-based cohort. Acta Obstetricia et Gynecologica Scandinavica. 2017;96(12):1475-83.

109. Griffin MP, Lake DE, Bissonette EA, Harrell FE, O'Shea TM, Moorman JR. Heart rate characteristics: novel physiomarkers to predict neonatal infection and death. Pediatrics. Nov 2005; 116(5):1070-4.

110. Singh A, Rasiah SV, Ewer AK. The impact of routine predischarge pulse oximetry screening in a regional neonatal unit. Arch Dis Child Fetal Neonatal Ed. Jul 2014;99(4):F297-302.

111. Aujard Y. 4 - Manifestations cliniques des infections néonatales: Clinical manifestations of neonatal infections. In: Aujard Y, editor. Infections néonatales. Paris: Elsevier Masson; 2015. p. 27-34.

112. Stevens DL, Stevens DL, Kaplan EL. Streptococcal Infections: Clinical Aspects, Microbiology, and Molecular Pathogenesis. Oxford University Press; 2000. 474 p.

113. Gaschignard J, Levy C, Romain O, Cohen R, Bingen E, Aujard Y, et al. Neonatal Bacterial Meningitis: 444 Cases in 7 Years. Pediatr Infect Dis J. March 2011;30(3):212-7.

114. Lin C, Chu S-M, Wang H-C, Yang P-H, Huang H-R, Chiang M-C, et al. Complicated Streptococcus agalactiae Sepsis with/without Meningitis in Young Infants and Newborns: The Clinical and Molecular Characteristics and Outcomes. Microorganisms. Oct 3, 2021;9(10):2094.

115. Zurina Z, Hoo NPJ, Amin-Nordin S, Joseph NMS, Nunis MA. Diagnosis of neonatal meningitis: is it time to use polymerase chain reaction? Med J Malaysia. Jan 2021;76(1):101-3.

116. Georget-Bouquinet E, Bingen E, Aujard Y, Levy C, Cohen R, Groupe des Pédiatres et Microbiologistes de l'Observatoire National des Méningites Bactériennes de l'Enfant. [Group B streptococcal meningitis'clinical, biological and evolutive features in children]. Arch Pediatr. Dec 2008;15 Suppl 3:S126-132.

117. Romain A-S, Cohen R, Plainvert C, Joubrel C, Béchet S, Perret A, et al. Clinical and Laboratory Features of Group B Streptococcus Meningitis in Infants and Newborns: Study of 848 Cases in France, 2001-2014. Clin Infect Dis. March 5, 2018;66(6):857-64.

118. Schmutz N, Henry E, Jopling J, Christensen RD. Expected ranges for blood neutrophil concentrations of neonates: the Manroe and Mouzinho charts revisited. J Perinatol. Apr 2008;28(4):275-81.

119. Hornik CP, Benjamin DK, Becker KC, Benjamin DK, Li J, Clark RH, et al. Use of the complete blood cell count in early-onset neonatal sepsis. Pediatr Infect Dis J. August 2012;31(8):799-802.

120. Andersen J, Christensen R, Hertel J. Clinical features and epidemiology of septicaemia and meningitis in neonates due to Streptococcus agalactiae in Copenhagen county, Denmark: a 10 year survey from 1992 to 2001. Acta Paediatrica. 2004;93(10):1334-9.

121. Jefferies AL. The management of term newborns at risk for early-onset bacterial sepsis. Paediatrics & Child Health. 1 Jul 2017;22(4):229-35.

122. Panda SK, Nayak MK, Rath S, Das P. The Utility of the Neutrophil-Lymphocyte Ratio as an Early Diagnostic Marker in Neonatal Sepsis. Cureus.

24 Jan 2021;13(1):e12891.

123. Thiery-Antier N, Binquet C, Vinault S, Meziani F, Boisramé-Helms J, Quenot J-P, et al. Is Thrombocytopenia an Early Prognostic Marker in Septic Shock? Crit Care Med. Apr 2016;44(4):764-72.

124. Jiang Z, Ye G-Y. 1:4 matched case-control study on influential factor of early onset neonatal sepsis. Eur Rev Med Pharmacol Sci. Sept 2013;17(18):2460-6.

125. Perrone S, Lotti F, Longini M, Rossetti A, Bindi I, Bazzini F, et al. C reactive protein in healthy term newborns during the first 48 hours of life. Arch Dis Child Fetal Neonatal Ed. March 2018;103(2):F163-6.

126. Mishra UK, Jacobs SE, Doyle LW, Garland SM. Newer approaches to the diagnosis of early onset neonatal sepsis. Arch Dis Child Fetal Neonatal Ed . May 2006;91(3):F208-12.

127. Oeser C, Pond M, Butcher P, Russell AB, Henneke P, Laing K, et al. PCR for the detection of pathogens in neonatal early onset sepsis. PLOS ONE. 24 Jan 2020;15(1):e0226817.

128. Hofer N, Zacharias E, Müller W, Resch B. An update on the use of C-reactive protein in early-onset neonatal sepsis: current insights and new tasks. Neonatology. 2012;102(1):25-36.

129. Eschborn S, Weitkamp J-H. Procalcitonin versus C-reactive protein: review of kinetics and performance for diagnosis of neonatal sepsis. J Perinatol. Jul 2019;39(7):893-903.

130. Ng PC. Diagnostic markers of infection in neonates. Arch Dis Child Fetal Neonatal Ed. May 2004;89(3):F229-235.

131. Nouri-Merchaoui S, Mahdhaoui N, Beizig S, Zakhama R, Fekih M, Methlouthi J, et al. Interest of serial C-reactive protein (CRP) in the management of newborns suspected of maternal-fetal bacterial infection: prospective study of 775 cases. Journal de pediatrie et de puericulture. 2009;2(22):80-8.

132. Franz AR, Steinbach G, Kron M, Pohlandt F. Reduction of Unnecessary Antibiotic Therapy in Newborn Infants Using Interleukin-8 and C-Reactive Protein as Markers of Bacterial Infections. Pediatrics. Sep 1, 1999;104(3):447-53.

133. Philip AG. Response of C-reactive protein in neonatal Group B streptococcal infection. Pediatr Infect Dis. Apr 1985;4(2):145-8.

134. Benitz WE. Adjunct laboratory tests in the diagnosis of early-onset neonatal sepsis. Clin Perinatol. June 2010;37(2):421-38.

135. Li X, Li T, Wang J, Feng Y, Ren C, Xu Z, et al. Clinical Value of C-Reactive Protein/Platelet Ratio in Neonatal Sepsis: A Cross-Sectional Study. J Inflamm

Res. 6 Oct 2021;14:5123-9.

136. Wang S-Y, Yu J-L. [Diagnostic value of procalcitonin in neonatal early-onset sepsis]. Zhongguo Dang Dai Er Ke Za Zhi. Apr 2020;22(4):316-22.

137. Puopolo KM, Benitz WE, Zaoutis TE, COMMITTEE ON FETUS AND NEWBORN, COMMITTEE ON INFECTIOUS DISEASES. Management of Neonates Born at ≤34 6/7 Weeks' Gestation With Suspected or Proven Early-Onset Bacterial Sepsis. Pediatrics. dec 2018;142(6):e20182896.

138. Altunhan H, Annagür A, Ors R, Mehmetoglu I. Procalcitonin measurement at 24 hours of age may be helpful in the prompt diagnosis of early-onset neonatal sepsis. Int J Infect Dis. Dec 2011;15(12):e854-858.

139. Chiesa C, Pacifico L, Osborn JF, Bonci E, Hofer N, Resch B. Early-Onset Neonatal Sepsis: Still Room for Improvement in Procalcitonin Diagnostic Accuracy Studies. Medicine (Baltimore). Jul 31, 2015;94(30):e1230.

140. Chiesa C, Natale F, Pascone R, Osborn JF, Pacifico L, Bonci E, et al. C reactive protein and procalcitonin: Reference intervals for preterm and term newborns during the early neonatal period. Clinica Chimica Acta. May 12, 2011;412(11):1053-9.

141. Guibourdenche J, Bedu A, Petzold L, Marchand M, Mariani-Kurdjian P, Hurtaud-Roux M-F, et al. Biochemical markers of neonatal sepsis: value of procalcitonin in the emergency setting. Ann Clin Biochem. March 2002;39(Pt 2):130-5.

142. Jost C, Mariani-Kurkdjian P, Biran V, Boissinot C, Bonacorsi S. Interest of perinatal sampling in the management of newborns suspected of early bacterial infections. Revue Francophone des Laboratoires. March 1, 2015;2015(470):43-53.

143. Sharma D, Farahbakhsh N, Shastri S, Sharma P. Biomarkers for diagnosis of neonatal sepsis: a literature review. J Matern Fetal Neonatal Med. June 2018;31(12):1646-59.

144. Bjornsdottir ES, Martins ER, Erlendsdottir H, Haraldsson G, Melo-Cristino J, Ramirez M, et al. Group B Streptococcal Neonatal and Early Infancy Infections in Iceland, 19762015. Pediatr Infect Dis J. 2019;38(6):620-4.

145. Guerti K, Devos H, Ieven MM, Mahieu LMY 2011. Time to positivity of neonatal blood cultures: fast and furious? Journal of Medical Microbiology;60(4):446-53.

146. Kumar Y, Qunibi M, Neal TJ, Yoxall CW. Time to positivity of neonatal blood cultures. Archives of Disease in Childhood - Fetal and Neonatal Edition. Nov 1, 2001;85(3):F182-6.

147. Jardine L, Davies MW, Faoagali J. Incubation time required for neonatal blood cultures to become positive. J Paediatr Child Health. Dec 2006;42(12):797-802.

148. Giannoni E, Agyeman PKA, Stocker M, Posfay-Barbe KM, Heininger U, Spycher BD, et al. Neonatal Sepsis of Early Onset, and Hospital-Acquired and Community-Acquired Late Onset: A Prospective Population-Based Cohort Study. J Pediatr. Oct 2018;201:106- 114.e4.

149. Garcia-Prats JA, Cooper TR, Schneider VF, Stager CE, Hansen TN. Rapid detection of microorganisms in blood cultures of newborn infants utilizing an automated blood culture system. Pediatrics. March 2000;105(3 Pt 1):523-7.

150. Connell TG, Rele M, Cowley D, Buttery JP, Curtis N. How Reliable Is a Negative Blood Culture Result? Volume of Blood Submitted for Culture in Routine Practice in a Children's Hospital. Pediatrics. May 1, 2007;119(5):891- 6.

151. Aujard Y, Bonacorsi S. 5 - Diagnostic biologique des infections néonatales: Biological diagnosis of neonatal infections. In: Aujard Y, editor. Infections néonatales. Paris: Elsevier Masson; 2015. p. 35-46.

152. Dagnew AF, Cunnington MC, Dube Q, Edwards MS, French N, Heyderman RS, et al. Variation in reported neonatal group B streptococcal disease incidence in developing countries. Clin Infect Dis. Jul 2012;55(1):91-102.

153. Sarkar SS, Bhagat I, Bhatt-Mehta V, Sarkar S. Does maternal intrapartum antibiotic treatment prolong the incubation time required for blood cultures to become positive for infants with early-onset sepsis? Am J Perinatol. March 2015;32(4):357-62.

154. Garges HP, Moody MA, Cotten CM, Smith PB, Tiffany KF, Lenfestey R, et al. Neonatal Meningitis: What Is the Correlation Among Cerebrospinal Fluid Cultures, Blood Cultures, and Cerebrospinal Fluid Parameters? Pediatrics. Apr 1, 2006;117(4):1094-100.

155. Srinivasan L, Harris MC, Shah SS. Lumbar Puncture in the Neonate: Challenges in Decision Making and Interpretation. Seminars in Perinatology. Dec 1, 2012;36(6):445-53.

156. Chemsi M, Elmasbahi F, Skali Lami A, Lehlimi M, Habzi A, Benomar S. Lumbar puncture in early bacterial neonatal infection: performance and decision. Journal de Pédiatrie et de Puériculture. March 1, 2018;31(1):27-33.

158. Stoll BJ, Hansen N, Fanaroff AA, Wright LL, Carlo WA, Ehrenkranz RA, et al. To Tap or Not to Tap: High Likelihood of Meningitis Without Sepsis Among Very Low Birth Weight Infants. Pediatrics. May 1, 2004;113(5):1181- 6.

159. Sturgeon JP, Zanetti B, Lindo D. C-Reactive Protein (CRP) levels in neonatal meningitis in England: an analysis of national variations in CRP cut-offs for lumbar puncture. BMC Pediatr. Dec 3, 2018;18(1):380.

160. Wang H, Zhu X. Cerebrospinal fluid culture-positive bacterial meningitis

increases the risk for neurologic damage among neonates. Ann Med;53(1):2199-204.

161. Kanegaye JT, Soliemanzadeh P, Bradley JS. Lumbar Puncture in Pediatric Bacterial Meningitis: Defining the Time Interval for Recovery of Cerebrospinal Fluid Pathogens After Parenteral Antibiotic Pretreatment. Pediatrics. Nov 1, 2001;108(5):1169-74.

162. Gordon SM, Srinivasan L, Harris MC. Neonatal Meningitis: Overcoming Challenges in Diagnosis, Prognosis, and Treatment with Omics. Frontiers in Pediatrics. 2017;5:139.

163. Rodriguez AF, Kaplan SL, Mason EO. Cerebrospinal fluid values in the very low birth weight infant. J Pediatr. June 1990;116(6):971-4.

164. Bonadio WA, Stanco L, Bruce R, Barry D, Smith D. Reference values of normal cerebrospinal fluid composition in infants ages 0 to 8 weeks. Pediatr Infect Dis J. July 1992;11(7):589-91.

165. Ansong AK, Smith PB, Benjamin DK, Clark RH, Li JS, Cotten CM, et al. Group B Streptococcal Meningitis: Cerebrospinal Fluid Parameters in the Era of Intrapartum Antibiotic Prophylaxis. Early Hum Dev. Oct 2009;85(10 Suppl):S5-7.

166. Neonatal infection (early onset): antibiotics for prevention and treatment | Guidance | NICE. NICE.

167. Deshmukh M, Mehta S, Patole S. Sepsis calculator for neonatal early onset sepsis - a systematic review and meta-analysis. J Matern Fetal Neonatal Med. June 2021;34(11):1832-40.

168. Gerdes JS. Diagnosis and management of bacterial infections in the neonate. Pediatr Clin North Am. August 2004;51(4):939-59, viii-ix.

169. Stocker M, Berger C, McDougall J, Giannoni E, Taskforce for the Swiss Society of Neonatology and the Paediatric Infectious Disease Group of Switzerland. Recommendations for term and late preterm infants at risk for perinatal bacterial infection. Swiss Med Wkly. 2013;143:w13873.

170. Dahesh S, Hensler ME, Van Sorge NM, Gertz RE, Schrag S, Nizet V, et al. Point mutation in the group B streptococcal pbp2x gene conferring decreased susceptibility to beta-lactam antibiotics. Antimicrob Agents Chemother. August 2008;52(8):2915-8.

171. Kekic D, Gajic I, Opavski N, Kojic M, Vukotic G, Smitran A, et al. Trends in molecular characteristics and antimicrobial resistance of group B streptococci: a multicenter study in Serbia, 2015-2020. Sci Rep. 12 Jan 2021;11:540.

172. Seki T, Kimura K, Reid ME, Miyazaki A, Banno H, Jin W, et al. High isolation rate of MDR group B streptococci with reduced penicillin susceptibility in Japan. J Antimicrob Chemother. oct 2015;70(10):2725-8.

173. Hayes K, O'Halloran F, Cotter L. A review of antibiotic resistance in Group B Streptococcus: the story so far. Crit Rev Microbiol. May 2020;46(3):253-69.

174. Back EE, O'Grady EJ, Back JD. High Rates of Perinatal Group B Streptococcus Clindamycin and Erythromycin Resistance in an Upstate New York Hospital. Antimicrob Agents Chemother. Feb 2012;56(2):739-42.

175. Campisi E, Rosini R, Ji W, Guidotti S, Rojas-Lopez M, Geng G, et al. Genomic Analysis Reveals Multi-Drug Resistance Clusters in Group B Streptococcus CC17 Hypervirulent Isolates Causing Neonatal Invasive Disease in Southern Mainland China. Front Microbiol. August 15, 2016;7:1265.

176. Mazzucchelli I, Garofoli F, Angelini M, Tinelli C, Tzialla C, Decembrino L. Rapid detection of bacteria in bloodstream infections using a molecular method: a pilot study with a neonatal diagnostic kit. Mol Biol Rep. Jan 2020;47(1):363-8.

177. Pammi M, Flores A, Versalovic J, Leeflang MM. Molecular assays for the diagnosis of sepsis in neonates. Cochrane Database Syst Rev. 1 Feb 2017;2:CD011926.

178. Edmond KM, Kortsalioudaki C, Scott S, Schrag SJ, Zaidi AKM, Cousens S, et al. Group B streptococcal disease in infants aged younger than 3 months: systematic review and meta-analysis. Lancet. Feb 11, 2012;379(9815):547-56.

179. Huang L, Gao K, Chen G, Zhong H, Li Z, Guan X, et al. Rapid Classification of Multilocus Sequence Subtype for Group B Streptococcus Based on MALDI-TOF Mass Spectrometry and Statistical Models. Front Cell Infect Microbiol. 2020;10:577031.

180. Koenig JM, Keenan WJ. Group B Streptococcus and Early-Onset Sepsis in the Era of Maternal Prophylaxis. Pediatr Clin North Am. June 2009;56(3):689- Contents.

181. Tazi A, Disson O, Bellais S, Bouaboud A, Tardieux I, Trieu-Cuot P, et al. Neonatal group B streptococcal meningitis - Identification of an essential virulence factor. Med Sci (Paris). Apr 1, 2011;27(4):362-4.

182. Leonidas JC, Hall RT, Beatty EC, Fellows RA. Radiographic findings in early onset neonatal group b streptococcal septicemia. Pediatrics. June 1977;59 Suppl(6 Pt 2):1006-11.

183. Vollman JH, Smith WL, Ballard ET, Light IJ. Early onset group B streptococcal disease: clinical, roentgenographic, and pathologic features. J Pediatr. August 1976;89(2):199-203.

184. Benomar S, Lahbabi MS, Belabbes H, El Mouatassim S, El Mdaghri N, Benbachir M. Neonatal group B streptococcal infection in Casablanca (Morocco). Médecine et Maladies Infectieuses. Dec 1 1998;28(12):932-6.

185. Yousef N. Lung ultrasound in the newborn. Archives of Pediatrics. March 1,

2016;23(3):317-21.

186. Ben Hamouda H, Ben Haj khalifa A, Hamza MA, Ayadi A, Soua H, Khedher M, et al. Clinical and evolutionary aspects of neonatal bacterial meningitis. Archives de Pédiatrie. Sep 1, 2013;20(9):938-44.

188. Chemsi M, Benomar S. Early neonatal bacterial infections. Journal of Pediatrics and Child Care. Feb 1, 2015;28(1):29-37.

189. Freitas FT de M, Romero GAS. Early-onset neonatal sepsis and the implementation of group B streptococcus prophylaxis in a Brazilian maternity hospital: a descriptive study. Braz J Infect Dis. Feb 2017;21(1):92-7.

190. Puopolo KM, Lynfield R, Cummings JJ, COMMITTEE ON FETUS AND NEWBORN, COMMITTEE ON INFECTIOUS DISEASES, Hand I, et al. Management of Infants at Risk for Group B Streptococcal Disease. Pediatrics. August 1, 2019;144(2):e20191881.

191. Malloy MH. Chorioamnionitis: epidemiology of newborn management and outcome United States 2008. J Perinatol. August 2014;34(8):611-5.

192. Brady MT, Polin RA. Prevention and management of infants with suspected or proven neonatal sepsis. Pediatrics. july 2013;132(1):166-8.

194. SFN. SFN, SFP, HAS 2017 _ Prise en charge du nouveau-né à risque d'infection néonatale bactérienne précoce (INBP) (≥ 34 SA) | Gynerisq.

195. Aujard Y, Bingen E. 8 - Méningites bactériennes néonatales: Neonatal bacterial meningitis. In: Aujard Y, editor. Infections néonatales. Paris: Elsevier Masson; 2015. p. 81-90.

196. Labenne M, Michaut F, Gouyon B, Ferdynus C, Gouyon J-B. A Population-Based Observational Study of Restrictive Guidelines for Antibiotic Therapy in Early-Onset Neonatal Infections. The Pediatric Infectious Disease Journal. July 2007;26(7):593-9.

197. Fjalstad JW, Stensvold HJ, Bergseng H, Simonsen GS, Salvesen B, Ronnestad AE, et al. Early-onset Sepsis and Antibiotic Exposure in Term Infants: A Nationwide Populationbased Study in Norway. Pediatr Infect Dis J. Jan 2016;35(1):1-6.

198. Leslibraires.fr. Intensive care and resuscitation of the newborn, POD - Guy Moriette, Michel Dehan, Francis Gold, Claud... - Elsevier Masson

199. Vergadi E, Manoura A, Chatzakis E, Karavitakis E, Maraki S, Galanakis E. Changes in the incidence and epidemiology of neonatal group B Streptococcal disease over the last two decades in Crete, Greece. Infect Dis Rep. Dec 5, 2018;10(3):7744.

200. Wynn JL, Polin RA. A neonatal sequential organ failure assessment score predicts mortality to late-onset sepsis in preterm very low birth weight infants.

Pediatr Res. July 2020;88(1):85-90.

201. Huang J, Lin X-Z, Lai J-D, Fan Y-F. [Group B streptococcus colonization in pregnant women and group B streptococcus infection in their preterm infants]. Zhongguo Dang Dai Er Ke Za Zhi. June 2019;21(6):567-72.

202. Grandgirard D, Leib SL. Meningitis in neonates: bench to bedside. Clin Perinatol. Sept 2010;37(3):655-76.

203. Bienenfeld S, Rodriguez-Riesco LG, Heyborne KD. Avoiding Inadequate Intrapartum Antibiotic Prophylaxis for Group B Streptococci. Obstet Gynecol. sept 2016;128(3):598-603.

204. Wynn JL. Defining neonatal sepsis. Curr Opin Pediatr. Apr 2016;28(2):135-40.

205. Bianchi-Jassir F, Paul P, To K-N, Carreras-Abad C, Seale AC, Jauneikaite E, et al. Systematic review of Group B Streptococcal capsular types, sequence types and surface proteins as potential vaccine candidates. Vaccine. 7 Oct 2020;38(43):6682-94.

206. Mukhopadhyay S, Puopolo KM, Hansen NI, Lorch SA, DeMauro SB, Greenberg RG, et al. Impact of Early-Onset Sepsis and Antibiotic Use on Death or Survival with Neurodevelopmental Impairment at 2 Years of Age among Extremely Preterm Infants. The Journal of Pediatrics. June 1, 2020;221:39-46.e5.

207. Horváth-Puhó E, Kassel MN van, Gonçalves BP, Gier B de, Procter SR, Paul P, et al. Mortality, neurodevelopmental impairments, and economic outcomes after invasive group B streptococcal disease in early infancy in Denmark and the Netherlands: a national matched cohort study. The Lancet Child & Adolescent Health. 1 June 2O21;5(6):398-407.

208. Nakwa FL, Lala SG, Madhi SA, Dangor Z. Neurodevelopmental Impairment at 1 Year of Age in Infants With Previous Invasive Group B Streptococcal Sepsis and Meningitis. Pediatr Infect Dis J. Sept 2020;39(9):794-8.

209. John HB, Arumugam A, Priya M, Murugesan N, Rajendraprasad N, Rebekah G, et al. South Indian children's neurodevelopmental outcomes after Group B Streptococcus invasive disease: A case cohort study. Clinical Infectious Diseases. Nov 3, 2021;(ciab792).

210. Kadambari S, Trotter CL, Heath PT, Goldacre MJ, Pollard AJ, Goldacre R. Group B Streptococcal Disease in England (1998 - 2017): A Population-based Observational Study. Clin Infect Dis. June 1, 2021;72(11):e791-8.

211. Ortgies T, Rullmann M, Ziegelhofer D, Blaser A, Thome UH. The role of early-onset- sepsis in the neurodevelopment of very low birth weight infants. BMC Pediatrics. June 25, 2021;21(1):289.

212. Schrag S, Gorwitz R, Fultz-Butts K, Schuchat A. Prevention of perinatal group B streptococcal disease. Revised guidelines from CDC. MMWR Recomm Rep. August 16, 2002;51(RR-11):1-22.

213. Bianchi-Jassir F, Seale AC, Kohli-Lynch M, Lawn JE, Baker CJ, Bartlett L, et al. Preterm Birth Associated With Group B Streptococcus Maternal Colonization Worldwide: Systematic Review and Meta-analyses. Clin Infect Dis. Nov 6, 2017;65(suppl_2):S133-42.

214. Hasperhoven G, Al-Nasiry S, Bekker V, Villamor E, Kramer B. Authors' reply re: Universal screening versus risk-based protocols for antibiotic prophylaxis during childbirth to prevent early-onset Group B streptococcal disease: a systematic review and meta-analysis. BJOG: An International Journal of Obstetrics & Gynaecology.
2020; 127(8):1039-40.

215. Nandyal RR. Update on group B streptococcal infections: perinatal and neonatal periods. J Perinat Neonatal Nurs. Sept 2008;22(3):230-7.

216. Li S, Huang J, Chen Z, Guo D, Yao Z, Ye X. Antibiotic Prevention for Maternal Group B Streptococcal Colonization on Neonatal GBS-Related Adverse Outcomes: A MetaAnalysis. Front Microbiol. 2017;8:374.

217. Vornhagen J, Adams Waldorf KM, Rajagopal L. Perinatal Group B Streptococcal Infections: Virulence Factors, Immunity, and Prevention Strategies. Trends Microbiol. nov 2017;25(11):919-31.

218. Hentgen V, Cohen R. [Maternal antibiotic use and Gram negative bacteria infection in neonates]. Arch Pediatr. nov 2012;19 Suppl 3:S135-139.

219. ACOG. Prevention of Group B Streptococcal Early-Onset Disease in Newborns: ACOG Committee Opinion Summary, Number 782. Obstet Gynecol. Jul 2019;134(1):1.

220. Amstey MS, Gibbs RS. Is penicillin G a better choice than ampicillin for prophylaxis of neonatal group B streptococcal infections? Obstet Gynecol. Dec 1994;84(6):1058-9.

221. Edwards RK, Clark P, Sistrom CL, Duff P. Intrapartum antibiotic prophylaxis 1: relative effects of recommended antibiotics on gram-negative pathogens. Obstet Gynecol. Sept 2002;100(3):534-9.

222. Canadian Paediatric Society. Management of term newborns at risk for early-onset bacterial sepsis | Canadian Paediatric Society.

223. Barber EL, Zhao G, Buhimschi IA, Illuzzi JL. Duration of intrapartum prophylaxis and concentration of penicillin G in fetal serum at delivery. Obstet Gynecol. August 2008;112(2 Pt 1):265-70.

224. Bizzarro MJ, Dembry L-M, Baltimore RS, Gallagher PG. Changing patterns in neonatal Escherichia coli sepsis and ampicillin resistance in the era of intrapartum antibiotic prophylaxis. Pediatrics. Apr 2008;121(4):689-96.

225. Seedat F, Brown CS, Stinton C, Patterson J, Geppert J, Freeman K, et al. Bacterial Load and Molecular Markers Associated With Early-onset Group B

Streptococcus: A Systematic Review and Meta-analysis. Pediatr Infect Dis J. 2018;37(12):e306-14.

226. Heyderman RS, Madhi SA, French N, Cutland C, Ngwira B, Kayambo D, et al. Group B streptococcus vaccination in pregnant women with or without HIV in Africa: a nonrandomised phase 2, open-label, multicentre trial. Lancet Infect Dis. May 2016;16(5):546-55.

227. Chen VL, Avci FY, Kasper DL. A maternal vaccine against group B Streptococcus: Past, present, and future. Vaccine. August 28, 2013;31:D13-9.

228. Lawn JE, Bianchi-Jassir F, Russell NJ, Kohli-Lynch M, Tann CJ, Hall J, et al. Group B Streptococcal Disease Worldwide for Pregnant Women, Stillbirths, and Children: Why, What, and How to Undertake Estimates? Clin Infect Dis. 6 Nov 2017;65(suppl_2):S89-99.

Appendices

Appendix 1: Protocol for the management of an asymptomatic newborn with suspected early bacterial neonatal infection ≥ 34SA (old protocol)

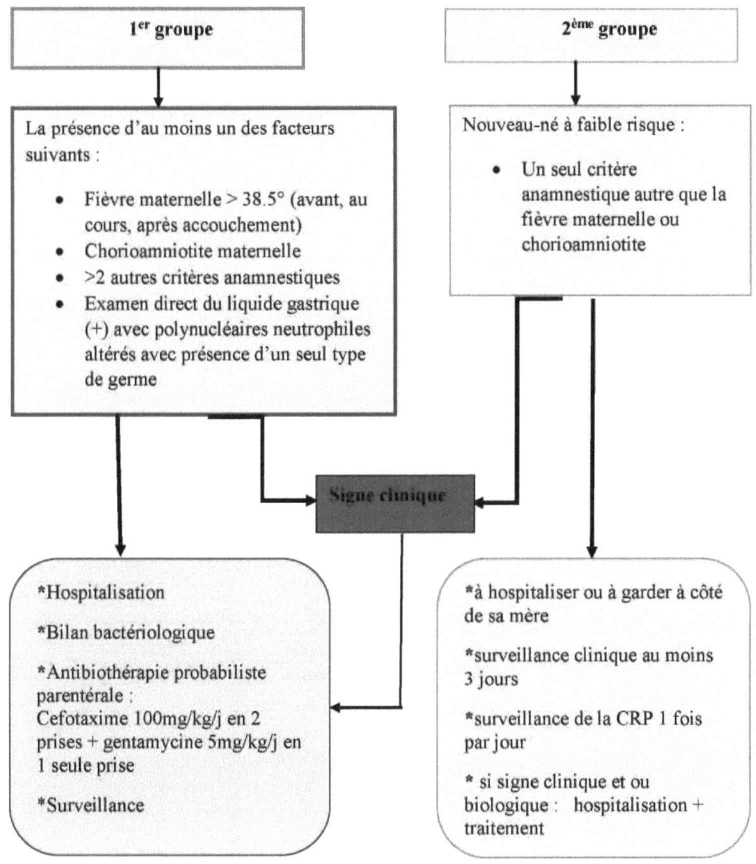

Appendix 2: Algorithm for management of an asymptomatic newborn
with suspected early bacterial neonatal infection ≥ 34 SA (new protocol)

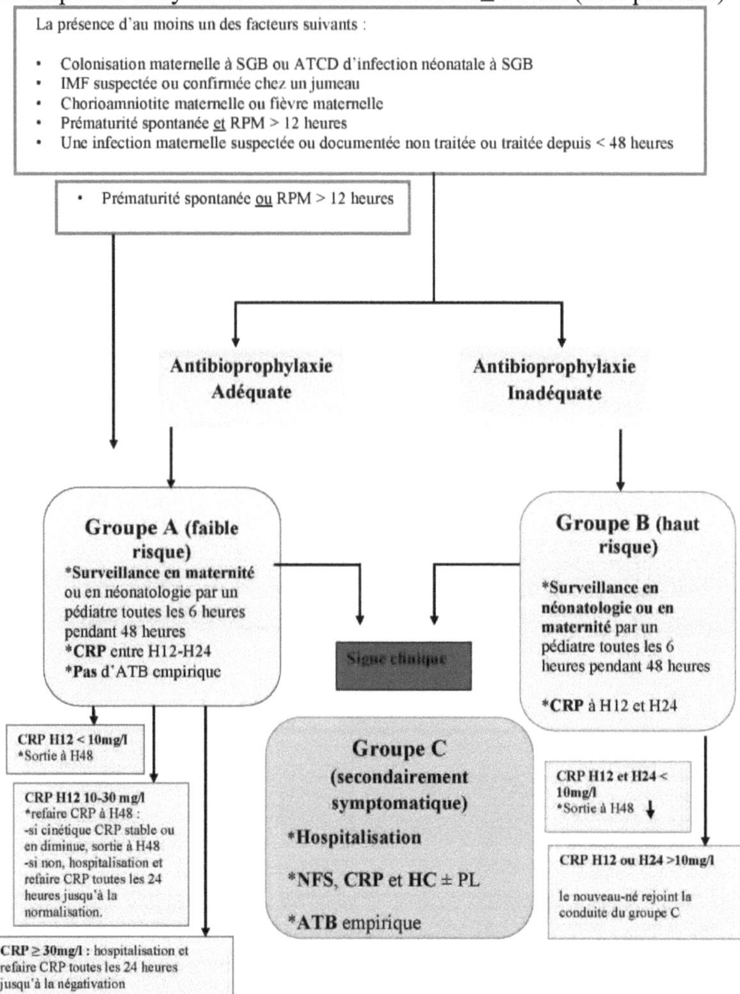

SUMMARY

Maternal-fetal infection with streptococcus B (or Streptococcus agalactiae) represents a major clinical challenge during pregnancy, for both mother and newborn. This pathogen, often present asymptomatically in the mother's genital tract, can be transmitted to the fetus during delivery, leading to serious complications such as neonatal sepsis, meningitis or pneumonia.

To prevent these complications, screening and prophylactic treatment strategies are crucial. Routine screening of pregnant women for streptococcus B, usually between the 35th and 37th weeks of pregnancy, can identify asymptomatic carriers. In the event of a positive test, intravenous antibiotic prophylaxis during labor is generally administered to reduce the risk of transmission to the newborn.

Proper management of this infection requires a multidisciplinary approach, involving obstetricians, pediatricians and infectious disease specialists, to ensure optimal care for both mother and baby. Patient education and awareness of the signs of postnatal infection are also essential to improve clinical outcomes.

In conclusion, although streptococcal B infection can lead to serious complications, screening and prophylactic treatment protocols have considerably reduced the risk to newborns. Continued vigilance and rigorous application of medical recommendations remain essential to ensure the health and well-being of mothers and babies.

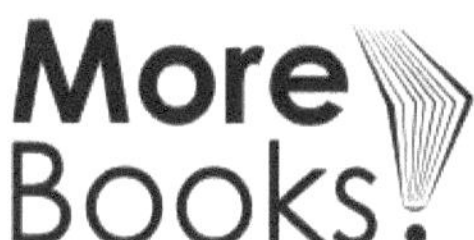
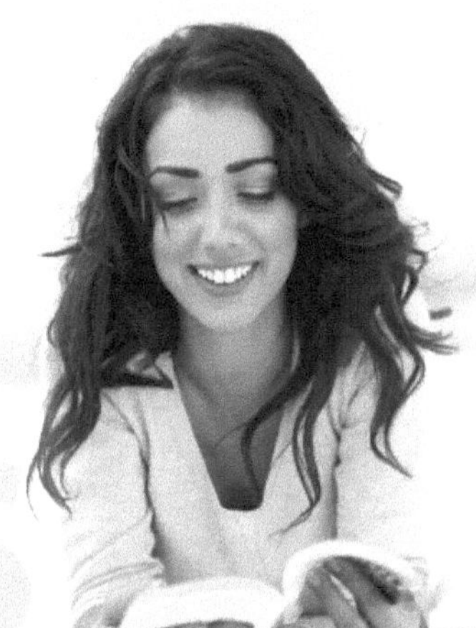

I want morebooks!

Buy your books fast and straightforward online - at one of world's fastest growing online book stores! Environmentally sound due to Print-on-Demand technologies.

Buy your books online at
www.morebooks.shop

Kaufen Sie Ihre Bücher schnell und unkompliziert online – auf einer der am schnellsten wachsenden Buchhandelsplattformen weltweit! Dank Print-On-Demand umwelt- und ressourcenschonend produzi ert.

Bücher schneller online kaufen
www.morebooks.shop

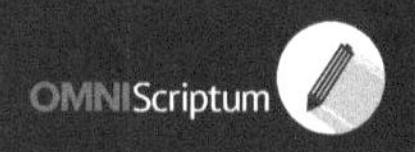